Lymphedema and Lipedema Nutrition Guide

foods, vitamins, minerals, and supplements

Chuck Ehrlich

Emily Iker, MD

Karen Louise Herbst, PhD, MD

Linda-Anne Kahn, CMT, CLT-LANA

Dorothy D. Sears, PhD

Mandy Kenyon, MS, RD, CSSD

Elizabeth McMahon, PhD

Foreword by Felicitie Daftuar

Lymph Notes
San Francisco

Lymphedema and Lipedema Nutrition Guide: foods, vitamins, minerals and supplements

Lymph Notes
2929 Webster Street
San Francisco, CA 94123 USA
www.LymphNotes.com   sales@lymphnotes.com

ISBN 978-0-9764806-8-6 paper; e-book 978-0-9764806-9-3
Library of Congress Control Number: 2015914637
Publishing history—first edition, printing 1-03

Cover image licensed from iStockPhoto. Some content and images adapted from Lymphedema Caregiver's Guide by permission of the publisher. Figure 4-1 images from www.fda.gov.

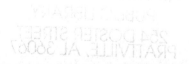

Table of Contents

Contents in Brief

Contents in Detail

Foreword

Four weeks after giving birth to my second child, I gained five pounds in five days, including a fat pad on the inside of my knee. I felt bloated and fatigued, with brain fog *far worse than post-partum sleep deprivation*. Looking back, I can say with confidence that my lipedema symptoms flared up due to a combination of salty seaweed soup, breastfeeding supplements, and postpartum hormones.

As president of the Lipedema Foundation and past president of the Fat Disorders Research Society, I've met hundreds of people with these conditions and heard many similar stories.

Diagnosis is a challenge if you go to your doctor and say that your legs are swollen, or heavy, or fat, or just plain weird. Fat disorders are different from obesity. Many people with lipedema are obese but there are also a lot of non-obese people. My doctor said the fat pad was simply post-partum depression. I was not depressed and pointed out that there was no way depression could cause that fat pad but, perhaps, it could work the other way around.

Some physicians say 'Stop eating' or 'Clean up your diet' to fix your legs. When we record everything we eat and go back to say, 'Here's my proof, I only eat 800 or 1,200 calories a day,' some will say 'Well, cut back another hundred calories.' That is not constructive. **Women can be obese with lipedema fat and anorexic at the same time.** In fact, I believe that eating too little only causes our bodies to store even more fat.

All too often, in the pursuit of better health, we venture outside the realm of the known and proven, only to get lost in the land of "What if..." and "Have you tried..." Wading through WebMD, research papers, advice of friends and specialists, blogs, and social media chatter is a circuitous and frustrating journey. Pick any health topic, search the Internet, and you will find multiple viewpoints—many in direct opposition to each other. In this book, a highly dedicated team summarizes the research and draws upon their experiences to help patients and caregivers change to a healthier eating pattern.

Nutrition does have a big impact on lipedema. For some people a simple change, such as giving up diet soda, makes a big difference in their pain and other lipedema symptoms. Other people find that lipedema pain diminishes, or goes away entirely, when switching to anti-inflammatory diets.

However, wading through the ever-evolving science of nutrition is difficult and confusing. Eggs, butter, dairy, gluten and grains have come in and out of favor. New oils and grains appear out of nowhere. What's a person to do?

Thanks to this experienced team, we have our answer. Tell your spouse and housemates that you need a few weeks of their patience while you make some changes and try a better way of eating. Grab your glasses of water and organic coffee, pull out your highlighters and pencils, put your feet up, and get reading. If you're short on time, skip straight to Chapter 3.

Felicitie Daftuar
Founder and Executive Director
Lipedema Foundation
www.lipedema.org

Preface

We wrote this book for people with lymphedema and lipedema because we believe nutrition is one of the most important aspects of self-care and treatment for these conditions.

Care providers have long recognized the importance of nutrition but been frustrated by a lack of specific guidelines and the difficulty of changing eating patterns. This guide addresses both issues based on our experience and the latest research.

Our team provides a variety of backgrounds and perspectives:

- Chuck Ehrlich is a medical researcher and writer for Lymph Notes, as well as a lymphedema caregiver.

- Emily Iker, MD, specializes in treating lymphedema and lipedema at the Lymphedema Center in Santa Monica and has lower-extremity lymphedema.

- Karen Louise Herbst, PhD, MD, treats people with lymphatic issues including lymphedema and lipedema, and leads the Treatment, Research and Education of Adipose Tissue (TREAT) Program, at the University of Arizona College of Medicine.

- Linda-Anne Kahn. CMT, NCTMB, CLT-LANA, CCN, is a lymphedema therapist, nutritional consultant and integrative health coach at Beauty Kliniek Day Spa and Wellness Center in San Diego, and has lipedema.

- Dorothy D. Sears, PhD, researches diet and behavior patterns for reducing disease risk at the University of California San Diego School of Medicine.

- Mandy Kenyon, MS, RD, CSSD, is a consulting dietitian and research leader for Salk Institute and Veteran's Medical Research Foundation.

- Elizabeth McMahon, PhD, is a clinical psychologist specializing in health-related behavior change and the author of several lymphedema books including **Overcoming the Emotional Challenges of Lymphedema**.

Emily Iker

I developed secondary lymphedema of the right leg following treatment for lymphoma, which interrupted my surgical residency. Consequently, I continued my studies in physical medicine and rehabilitation. After completing my residency at New York Medical College, I moved to Los Angeles and assisted an orthopedic surgeon for several years before opening my own practice.

Frustrated by the lack of lymphedema treatment options, I started the Lymphedema Center in Santa Monica in 1994. In 1995, I received my Certification of Lymphedema Management from Prof. Albert Leduc, the world-renowned lymphologist. My center is dedicated to diagnosing and managing lymphedema and lipedema. I am actively involved in patient education, research, and raising awareness of these conditions through organizations such as LE&RN. I lecture and teach on national and international level.

For me, lymphedema self-care is both routine and a challenge, especially when I am travelling. I am very careful to maintain my daily routine including skin care, self-massage, exercises, and compression, as well as maintaining healthy organic diet.

Linda-Anne Kahn

Growing up in South Africa, I was very active in sports including field hockey, swim team (I trained and swam 6 miles daily), exercise classes, and trampoline. I rode my bicycle to school every day.

I noticed that I didn't have ankles like the other girls. I hated my "thick" ankles especially in my school uniform with socks and laced shoes, which made my ankles look even worse. As I became a teenager, my legs became larger and I became so self-conscious. I had a small waist and flat stomach and larger legs. One day my aunt remarked that I had the family thighs and I never wore shorts again. My grandmother and two aunts had "heavy legs" and we just thought that was how we were in my family.

In my teens, I began dieting and jogging daily, weighing my food, and some-times not eating properly for days in an attempt to reduce my legs. My waist got smaller and my arms became skinny but my legs stayed the same. I began yo-yo dieting, which lasted for years. In college, I put on 20 pounds and felt awful. When I was in my 20's I was almost anorexic, took diet pills, and tried hard not to eat too much. Prior to my menstrual period, my legs would ache. I hated my legs!

I began noticing that certain foods, like bread and cheese, made me bloat terribly so I eliminated those foods. During my first pregnancy, I was very careful and I only put on 18 pounds. Two years later, I became pregnant again and put on 40 pounds, which was very difficult to get rid of.

When I was 30 years old, I immigrated to the United States. It was a very stressful time and I began eating Baskin Robbins ice cream, cream cheese, bagels, pasta, chocolate, and processed foods and I put on 25 pounds. It was a struggle and my weight fluctuated daily. I could put on 5 pounds overnight. I was bloated, tired, constipated, uncomfortable and not happy with my body. My stomach looked as though I was 3 month pregnant after eating. I then became vegan for 12 years, but ate so much brown rice, beans and starchy items that I put on weight.

Then I began studying nutrition and realized that I could not eat any bread or pasta. I finally settled on a diet with some fish, vegetable juices, some fruit, moderate grains (wild rice, brown rice), and legumes and my weight began stabilizing. I tried the raw food diet and cleansing and could lose 8 pounds in a week, but it would come back with a few weeks, once going back to regular eating.

In 1991 at the Dr. Vodder School in Austria, my beloved lymphedema therapy teacher Hildegard Wittlinger diagnosed me with stage 1 lipedema. With new knowledge of my condition, I began searching for the missing link and putting together an anti-inflammatory diet.

Hildegard told us about small chain fatty acids being important for lipedema, as these fats bypass the small intestine and can be helpful to lipedema patients. I discovered coconut oil and began incorporating that into my diet. I went on a three week cleanse every year, began eliminating the inflammatory foods and for the first time in my life I enjoyed my food. I became a wonderful cook! I incorporated dry brushing, lymphatic massage, and deep breathing exercises into my daily routine.

My present exercise routine is Pilates twice a week, yoga once a week and walking every day. I am 3 pants sizes smaller than I was 25 years ago. I am dairy free, gluten free, sugar free and do not eat red meat, chicken or turkey. In recent months, I have incorporated goat kefir onto my diet. I eat fermented foods, vegetables, and low glycemic fruits daily, as well as eggs, quinoa, brown rice, and wild salmon, when available. I avoid GMO foods and only eat organic foods at home.

At 66 years old, I am more energetic and vital than ever before. For the first time in my life, I am not unhappy with my body. My stomach is flat most of the time and I do not bloat after meals. I did not progress to stage 2 lipedema and I continue to feel better, with high energy and acceptance of my "lippy" legs, which look much better than they did before. Recently I was so excited to fit into my favorite tight jeans that I had saved for over 25 years.

Lipedema is treatable and I love sharing and coaching my patients on a path to optimal health.

Introduction

Eating to Starve Lymphedema and Lipedema

You can starve lymphedema and lipedema by eating foods that fight these conditions and avoiding foods that make them worse. Benefits of better food choices include:

- Improving your symptoms, overall health, and quality of life.

- Delaying changes associated with progression to more advanced stages.

- Reducing your risk of developing symptoms, for those at risk.

Starving these conditions does not mean that you go hungry. We recommend a wide variety of tasty and satisfying foods, without limiting portions.

'Eating to starve' comes from a TED Talk by William Li on dietary cancer prevention. His research into foods that fight tumor growth validated our thinking about using foods to combat disease and supports our recommended 'fighting foods.' Eating to starve cancer overlaps with our work because cancer causes lymphedema and shares many underlying mechanisms. We also looked at food for fighting other conditions that contribute to lymphedema or lipedema—such as liver disease, cardiovascular disease, and diabetes—and incorporated them into our recommendations.

Our goal is to help you feel better and improve your health by changing what you eat. This guide is also for health care professionals, family, and friends who want to learn more about lymphedema, lipedema, and the latest nutrition research.

We view nutrition as an essential part of treatment for lymphedema and lipedema, with the same importance as the traditional pillars of Complex Decongestive Therapy (CDT): skin care, compression, lymphatic drainage, and exercise.

Nutrition alone is not adequate treatment, but many people will gain little benefit from CDT without changing their eating pattern. Lymphedema caused by obesity can be improved or even reversed with better nutrition. Although much of what we think about the influence of nutrition on disease is based on inference (in the absence of objective data), this information is still useful and important.

Proper nutrition is a life-long concern and should start with prenatal nutrition and continue through infancy and childhood. Childhood obesity has many undesirable effects including abnormally elevated levels of undesirable estrogen metabolites in girls, prior to starting puberty [1] and significantly increased risk of liver disease in both sexes [2].

How to Use This Book

Use this guide to understand what foods to eat, why, and how to prepare them:

- Chapter 1 will help you understand lymphedema and lipedema in more detail including signs and symptoms and how these conditions change at different stages.

- Chapter 2 summarizes the research supporting our food recommendations in terms of relevant physical processes (physiology) and the ways in which food choices affect these processes.

- Chapter 3 summarizes our recommended eating pattern in terms of foods to eat routinely and foods to avoid or eat infrequently.

- Chapters 4 and 5 explain important nutrients and nutritional factors in foods including nutrients identified on food labels and other important nutritional factors.

- Chapter 6 covers vitamins, minerals and supplements, including some that anyone with lymphedema or lipedema should consider taking.

- Chapter 7 guides you through the process of changing your eating pattern by providing tools for decision making, helping you build support, identifying and obtaining missing skills, sustaining change, coping with emotional issues, dealing with difficult situations, etc.

- Chapter 8 provides example meal plans and menus, as well as suggestions for menu planning and changing tastes.

- Chapter 9 includes a variety of healthy recipes for all occasions.

- Chapter 10 provides instructions on preparing different vegetables and fruits.

- Chapter 11 contains practical tips for including healthier alternatives to favorite foods and tips for eating away from home.

- Chapter 12 covers record keeping in support of change and problem solving.

- Appendix A is our suggested shopping guide.

- Appendix B is the list of ingredients to avoid.

- Appendix C includes risk factors for developing lymphedema or lipedema, factors that distinguish between these conditions, and information on treatment and other health care considerations.

- Appendix D has photos of people with lymphedema and lipedema in all stages of each condition and combinations of lymphedema and lipedema.

- Appendix E contains a list of resources and sources of additional information.

Is Lipedema Lymphedema?

Lipedema, or painful fat syndrome, is an inherited chronic disease condition, as explained later. We consider lipedema to be a form of lymphedema and a vascular disorder as well as a fat disorder. Although we use both terms, almost everything we say about lymphedema applies to lipedema.

Previously thinking was that lipedema caused lymphedema only in the later stages of the condition when visible swelling develops, especially in the feet. We now know that abnormal increased tissue fluid from leaky blood and lymphatic vessels contributes to abnormal fat accumulation in early stage lipedema, even though swelling (edema) is not apparent.

Your Mileage May Vary

We know from experience that people can respond differently to foods or supplements and many factors influence how foods make you feel and support your health. Certain factors are fixed (like genetics), some factors change over time (like your age), some can be changed intentionally (such as your eating pattern), and some unexpected events have effects (like infections requiring antibiotics).

Please use our recommendations as guidelines and work with your health care team to discover an eating pattern that works for you, at this time in your life. We provide tools to help you find the eating pattern that supports your health and fits your lifestyle.

Focus on moving to a healthy eating pattern that you can enjoy and sustain. Avoid major short-term changes in your eating pattern, unless there is a medical reason.

Adapt our food recommendations to your own tastes and food preferences. Skip any foods or supplements that may trigger food allergies, food sensitivities, digestive disorders, histamine intolerance, etc.

If you are being treated for cancer, or have recently completed treatment, ask your care team about consulting a registered dietitian for nutritional recommendations tailored to your condition and treatment. The American Cancer Society also provides information on nutrition during and after treatment; see www.cancer.org.

If you have had weight loss surgery, gastric bypass surgery, other gastrointestinal surgery, or if you have a medical condition of the gastrointestinal tract or metabolism (such as diabetes), please coordinate changing your eating pattern with your health care team.

Let Us Know What Works

Please keep in touch to let us know what works for you and how we can improve this book. E-mail is best: nutrition@lymphnotes.com. Errata and lessons learned will be shared on the book website (www.lymphnotes.com/nutrition.php).

Never Say Diet

You may notice that we generally avoid the term 'diet.' This is because we want to help you to find an eating pattern that helps you feel better and you can enjoy for the foreseeable future. Consistently following a healthy eating pattern is better for you physically and emotionally than bouncing between diets that you cannot sustain long term.

Chapter 1

Lymphedema and Lipedema

Signs and symptoms of lymphedema and lipedema include increasing swelling (edema), fat accumulation, skin changes, and increased risk of infection (cellulitis, wounds, or ulcers) in affected areas, as explained below.

Lymphedema and lipedema are chronic progressive conditions that can become painful, depressing, disfiguring, disabling, and (potentially) deadly, without treatment. Treatment and self-care (including nutrition) relieves pain and other symptoms, and can slow the progression of these conditions. See Appendix C for more information on diagnosis, treatment and other health care considerations.

Early recognition, diagnosis, and treatment provide the best results. Follow-up with your health care provider if you think you have lymphedema or lipedema but have not been diagnosed.

If you have one or more risk factors for developing these conditions (see Appendix C), following our recommended eating pattern may help reduce your risk. Remain alert to potential signs and symptoms and follow up with your health care provider, especially if a tissue infection is your first sign of lymphedema.

Signs and Symptoms

Signs and symptoms of lymphedema and lipedema include:

- Skin or tissue infection (cellulitis) or a history of infection, can be a sign, or the first sign, of lymphedema because these infections are rare in normal skin. If you are at risk for lymphedema, seek medical care immediately if you have signs of a skin infection: localized redness, warmth, raised areas, body ache, malaise, increased joint pain, fever, chills, etc.

- Persistent swelling (edema) that does not go away with rest or elevation and lacks a known cause, such as a sprain or other injury. Swelling may start near the trunk of the body (proximal) or at the distant end of a limb (distal) depending on the causes.

- Skin color is generally normal for swelling from lymphedema or lipedema; if the swollen area is red, angry, itchy, or hot, that may indicate an infection. Multi-color bruising indicates an injury; dark stains on swollen areas indicate blood leakage from venous disease and phlebolymphedema.

- Legs or thighs that are symmetrically larger or heavy (at least initially), and out of proportion with the upper body, are characteristics of lipedema. Leg swelling from lymphedema is not usually symmetric.

- Cankles or unusually thick ankles can be signs of either lymphedema or lipedema. Lymphedema starts with swelling that becomes fat, includes the toes, and is rarely symmetric; lipedema fat on the legs is symmetric and stops at the ankles initially (see the photos in Appendix D) and does not involve the feet until advanced stages (Stage 4).

- Arm fat accumulation that is symmetrical on both upper arms (biceps or triceps) can also be lipedema. See the photos in Appendix D for examples.

- Abdominal fat and swelling (belly fat) can expand to form a hanging flap or apron (abdominal panniculus).

- Swelling or fat in the trunk or genitals.

- Painful fat that is tender to touch and bruises easily is characteristic of lipedema.

- Feeling of aching or heaviness in the at-risk limb, even before there is noticeable swelling.

- Rings, bracelets, sleeves, socks, or shoes that suddenly feel too tight or do not fit.

- Lipedema fat may initially (very early stage) look and feel exceptionally soft and smooth, like butter. As lipedema progresses, fat cells become progressively larger and the skin no longer feels smooth; in later stages visible nodules (cellulite) cause the skin to look and feel dimpled or lumpy and fatty protrusions may develop.

- Wounds or ulcers that are unusually slow to heal or not healing.

Skin changes in areas affected by lymphedema may include:

- Swollen skin that initially feels soft or watery and will indent if pressed (pitting edema). Stretch marks may appear on the stretched skin.

- Saggy loose skin, following a reduction in swelling. For example, during intensive lymphedema treatment.

- Stiffer, gel-like, and lumpy skin due to protein build-up during the early stages of fibrosis.

- Hard, leathery, or scaly skin from continued protein build-up and advanced fibrosis.

- Red and inflamed skin that has stretched to accommodate extra fluid.

- Blisters from fluid buildup and watery fluid escaping from openings in the skin (weeping lymphedema, or lymphorrhea).

- Orange peel appearance (*peau d'orange*) of thickened skin with congested lymph vessels.

- Warty growths (papillomas), especially on the legs.

See Appendix C for the factors that distinguish lymphedema from lipedema and photos showing examples of these conditions in Appendix D.

Lymphedema

Lymphedema results when the lymphatic system is overloaded, damaged, or defective. The lymphatic system helps fight infections and cancer, removes cellular waste, maintains fluid balance and controls blood pressure, and processes fats from foods. These functions are impaired in someone with lymphedema.

Lymphatic vessels are found near arteries and veins throughout the body. Tiny lymphatic collectors remove excess tissue fluid from the spaces between cells in the skin, the gut, and around other organs. This lymphatic fluid, or lymph, flows through a network of lymph nodes and progressively larger lymphatic vessels and trunks before emptying into the blood circulatory system at the base of the neck. Lymph nodes monitor the fluid for signs of infection, break down harmful microbes, and concentrate the fluid by

Stages of Lymphedema
The International Society of Lymphology (ISL) staging system uses stages 0 to III [**3**].
• Stage 0 (or Ia): a latent or sub-clinical condition where swelling is not yet evident despite impaired lymph drainage, subtle changes in tissue fluid composition, and changes in subjective symptoms. It may exist months or years before overt edema occurs (Stages I-III).
• Stage I represents an early accumulation of fluid relatively high in protein content (in comparison with venous edema) which subsides with limb elevation. Pitting may occur. An increase in various proliferating skin cells may also be seen.
• Stage II signifies that limb elevation alone rarely reduces tissue swelling and pitting is seen. Late in Stage II, the limb may or may not pit as excess fat and fibrosis replaces swelling.
• Stage III includes lymphostatic elephantiasis where pitting can be absent and abnormal skin changes such as thickening and pigment changes, further deposition of fat and fibrosis, and warty overgrowths have developed.
See the photos of each stage in Appendix D.

removing excess water.

Lymphatic vessels contain segments with one-way valves at each end (lymphangions). Segments contract periodically, creating a pumping motion that pushes fluid into the next segment along the vessel. Fluid overload stretches the lymphatic vessels, causing one-way valves to fail, interfering with pumping, and allowing reverse flow (backflow) that increases dependent edema.

Lymphedema is characterized by swelling (edema) from excess tissue fluid trapped in the skin and tissues. Over time, stagnant fluid causes skin changes, fat accumulation, and progression to more advanced stages. In some cases, excess lymph may leak through the skin (weeping lymphedema) or accumulate in the abdomen (ascites).

Types of Lymphedema

There are two types of lymphedema, primary and secondary, based on different causes, although the cause may not be clear. These types are not exclusive; a person may have both because primary lymphedema increases the risk of secondary lymphedema. Treatment and care are the same for both types.

Primary lymphedema results from congenital lymphatic system defects that interfere with fluid removal. Swelling or other signs of lymphedema may be noticeable at birth, during infancy or appear around puberty, during pregnancy, or later in life. Inheritable genetic factors have been linked to certain types of primary lymphedema.

Secondary lymphedema results from lymphatic system damage or overload. Common causes of secondary lymphedema include cancer treatment, other trauma or injury, obesity, congestive heart failure, chronic venous insufficiency, lipedema, diabetes, etc.

Phlebolymphedema

One of the most common forms of secondary lymphedema in older people is phlebolymphedema, a combination of lymphedema and chronic venous insufficiency (CVI). Venous and lymphatic insufficiency results in swelling of the lower legs and feet. Reddish-brown skin discoloration and hyperpigmentation (hemosiderin staining) are common signs of venous involvement. See the photos in Appendix D.

Lipedema

Lipedema, or painful fat syndrome, is characterized by excess fat developing below the waist and extending down to the ankles but stopping above the feet. About 80% of cases involve both legs and arms; only 3% are arms only. The fat is symmetric (in the early stages), tender, often painful, and bruises easily.

Types of lipedema are defined based on the affected areas (see "Types of Lipedema" on page 21 and the photos in Appendix D). Lipedema can develop along with lymphedema, obesity, or other less common adipose tissue disorders, such as Dercum's disease or multiple symmetric lipomatosis.

Characteristics that distinguish lipedema from lymphedema include:

- Pain: lipedema patients often complain of pain when touched; particularly on the legs. For example, when their cat walks on them.

- Bruising and subcutaneous bleeding may occur from impact or spontaneously.

- Tissues affected by lipedema alone are not prone to the infections that characterize lymphedema. Infections are more likely after lymphedema swelling develops.

- In the early stages of lipedema, the upper part of the body may remain slim while fat accumulates from the tops of the hips to the ankles without involving the feet [5]. The feet are spared, swelling stops at the ankles, and a skin-fold test (Stemmer sign) on the top of the foot or toes is negative.

- Weight gain accumulates evenly on the affected areas on both legs from the top of the hip down to the ankle. Leg fat from lipedema appears more symmetric than swelling from lymphedema.

- Weight loss comes only from areas that are not affected by lipedema. There may be weight loss from the legs if lipedema is combined with obesity.

- Swelling in the legs usually gets worse after standing, during times of increased heat, and during the second half of the day. Some individuals experience reduced swelling during sleep; others do not experience this benefit.

Dercum's Disease and Multiple Symmetric Lipomatosis

Dercum's disease (adiposis dolorosa) is characterized by very painful nodular subcutaneous adipose tissue (SAT) and other signs and symptoms that typically develop around the age of 35 (although Dercum's can occur in children and older individuals). Clinically people with Dercum's disease can look like they have lipedema or familial multiple lipomatosis. The pain is chronic, can move around, is often disabling, and resistant to traditional analgesics. Associated symptoms include easy bruising, gastrointestinal complaints, joint and muscle pain, sleep disturbances, impaired memory, depression, difficulty concentrating, anxiety, rapid heartbeat, shortness of breath, diabetes, bloating, constipation, fatigue, weakness and joint aches.

Multiple symmetric lipomatosis (MSL) is a rare syndrome characterized by the painless, symmetrical accumulation of abnormal tumor-like SAT, either as discrete non-encapsulated lipomas or as a flowing increase in SAT. The appearance and location of SAT in MSL can vary. Individuals with MSL have increased SAT in a symmetrical distribution on the neck, the back, the chest, the upper arms, or on the thighs. MSL usually spares the extremities but altered fat may involve the whole body. Fat and muscle wasting can occur in other areas [4].

- Lipedema skin is smooth initially but over time, fatty lumps called nodules develop within the affected tissues and the skin appears lumpy.

- In the later stages of lipedema, larger, rounded, fat deposits called lobules develop making legs irregularly shaped and interfering with posture and walking.

Lipedema is rarely seen in Asian women. Lipedema in men is very rare and may be linked to abnormal hormone levels or liver disease.

Lipedema typically appears during puberty and increases during pregnancy or menopause. Changes in body shape from lipedema can start before puberty and lipedema fat on legs and arms may be apparent by the age of eight. One pediatric clinic reported that 6.5% of patients referred for lymphedema

Stages of Lipedema

Lipedema progresses through these stages:

- Stage 1: Normal skin surface with enlarged areas of fat.

- Stage 2: Uneven skin with indentations in the fat (cellulite), the surface of the skin takes on the lumpy appearance of a mattress with fat globules bulging between thickened connective fibers (fibrotic septa).

- Stage 3: Large extrusions of tissue causing deformations especially on the thighs and around the knees.

- Stage 4: Lipedema with lymphedema (lipolymphedema); abnormal fat on the hands, feet, trunk and head.

Photos of each stage are in Appendix D.

actually had lipedema [7].

In very early stage lipedema, the skin in affected areas looks normal and the fat is very smooth and soft. Over time, the fat becomes increasingly nodular. When lipedema progresses to more advanced stages, the rectangular compartments of fat and connective tissue below the skin become larger and protrude, causing a mattress-like appearance that can include larger fatty lumps (lipomas). Fat on the inner legs can form lobules that restrict mobility and damage the knees and other joints.

Lipedema fat alone does not harm the heart or metabolism as does abdominal fat. Women can have large amounts of lipedema fat and be considered obese, yet remain metabolically healthy if they avoid abdominal obesity.

Although lipedema is an inherited condition, the specific genes involved have not been identified. Inheritance appears to be autosomal dominant, passing from mother or father to daughter.

Lipedema causes visible lymphedema swelling in the later stages and swelling may extend into the feet. The combined condition is lipolymphedema [8]. Lymphedema care recommendations apply to both conditions.

Types of Lipedema

European Lymphology Society sub-classification system for types of lipedema based on segments of the lower body affected allows for a mixture of types in a given individual [6]:

- Type I: buttock and hips (saddle bag phenomena).

- Type II: buttock to knees.

- Type III: buttock to ankles.

- Type IV: arms and legs affected.

- Type V: lipolymphedema.

One characteristic of lipedema is persistent enlargement of the hips, buttocks and legs. Fat in these areas remains unaffected by weight loss efforts involving diet, exercise, weight loss medications, or weight loss surgery, even though weight is lost from unaffected areas, usually the trunk.

Chapter 2

Physiology and Food Choices

Lymphedema and lipedema cause swelling, inflammation, and fat accumulation in the skin but they are not skin conditions. They involve multiple body systems and are linked to multiple medical conditions.

In terms of eating to starve these conditions, the interesting body systems include:

- Gut lymphatics: a major source of lymph.

- Gut microbes: an internal ecosystem important to your health.

- Grains and gluten metabolism: how common foods can elicit dysfunction and disease.

- Liver: another major source of lymph.

- Skin: a multi-function organ.

- Abnormal biological signals: how tumors and other conditions promote lymphedema.

- Lipedema fat: unique properties and the role of estrogen.

We describe the role of food choices in each system to help you understand your condition and the reasoning behind our recommendations. The relative importance of each system to your health depends upon your symptoms, and may change over time.

Gut Lymphatics

Although lymphedema care focuses on the skin, most of the lymphatic system is deeper inside the body. Networks of lymphatic vessels and lymph nodes surround the internal organs, especially the digestive organs and the heart.

Lymphatics in the gut (gut associated lymphoid tissues or GALT) make up 70% of the immune system. Gut lymphatics monitor digestive tract contents for harmful elements and provide the first line of defense against foodborne infections, as well as helping with fat metabolism and other functions.

The lymphatic system so delicate that damage or overload in one area can affect lymph flow in distant parts of the network. Lymph moves more slowly and at lower pressures than blood, which is pumped by the heart. Lymph is propelled by lymphatic vessel contractions, movement of skeletal muscles surrounding lymphatic vessels (muscle pump), deep breathing that flexes the diaphragm and pumps the central lymphatic vessels (cisterna chyli), and small pressure differences between lymphatic vessels.

Over half of all lymph originates from the gut under normal conditions. Liver disease (see "Fatty Liver Disease" on page 41) or high-dietary fat intake can produce from 2 to 10 times the normal lymph volume, overloading the central lymphatic vessels, and contributing to swelling in other parts of the body.

Increased lymph volume from the gut, especially when combined with lymphatic vessel leakage (discussed below), affects all parts of the body:

- Arm, head, or neck swelling can increase due to central lymphatic congestion.

- Abdominal fat and swelling (abdominal edema or lymph belly) increase and can form a hanging flap (abdominal panniculus).

- Genital swelling (genital edema).

- Leg swelling when overload damages the one-way valves in the lymphatic vessels, lymph from the gut can flow into the legs (backflow), driven by increased lymphatic pressure and assisted by gravity.

- Lymph leaking through the skin (weeping lymphedema or lymphorrhea) of the trunk or legs.

- Lymph backflow into other body spaces (chylous reflux and ascites) in extreme cases.

Gut Lymphatics and Chyle

The walls of the small intestine contain two networks of lymphatic vessels. One removes excess tissue fluid from the intestine itself and the other collects fats from food being digested in the small intestine in the form of chyle, a milky white fluid.

Fat entering the small intestine from the stomach triggers the release of bile from the gallbladder into the small intestine. Bile separates triglycerides into one sugar (glycerol) and three fatty acid molecules. Fats from foods are primarily long-chain fats but certain foods mostly short- and medium-chain fats as explained in Chapter 4. Sugars and short- or medium-chain fats are absorbed into blood vessels in the wall of the small intestine.

Long-chain fats and cholesterol from foods are absorbed by enterocyte cells on the surface of tiny, finger-like projections (intestinal villi) that line the small intestine. Within the villi, fats move from the enterocytes into special lymphatic vessels (lacteals) as chylomicrons and accumulate into a milky liquid called chyle.

Chyle flows through lymphatic vessels surrounding the small intestine, into a collecting vessel (cisterna chyli) located just below the diaphragm, and then into the central lymphatic vessels (thoracic duct), which empties into the bloodstream at the base of the neck (left subclavian vein). The blood delivers fats from the chyle (triglycerides) to fat and muscle tissues throughout the body, and cholesterol to the liver [9].

Intestinal fat absorption is impaired by lymphatic system defects in some types of congenital lymphedema. Children with these conditions have digestive problems and risk malnutrition because they cannot metabolize long-chain fats.

Lymphatic vessel blockage or chyle leakage can result in the loss of protein, fat-soluble vitamins, and electrolytes, possibly leading to acidosis and impaired immune function. Symptoms of chyle leakage vary and may include nonspecific discomfort, respiratory distress or abdominal distention [10].

Failure of the lymphatic system to absorb fats or transport chyle can trigger subcutaneous edema, chylous ascites, chylothorax, or chylous reflux. Excess chyle also contributes to cardiovascular disease, obesity, chronic inflammation, and metabolic syndrome [11].

Food Choices and Chyle Volume

Foods contain different mixtures of fat types, depending on the type of food (as explained in Chapter 4). Long-chain fats are by far the most common and are converted into chyle and processed through the lymphatic system. Short- and medium-chain fats are less common and are not converted to chyle. These fats are absorbed into the bloodstream by capillaries in the small intestine and passed to the liver via the portal vein with other nutrients.

Excessive long-chain fat intake can double the volume of chyle produced in the intestine and add an extra half gallon (2 liters) of fluid to the lymphatic system every day [12].

Eating to Starve Chyle Volume

Feed healthy metabolism with medium- and short-chain fats that pass directly from the small intestine into the liver via the bloodstream:

- MCT oil (medium chain-triglyceride oil) derived from coconuts, coconut oil, and other coconut foods are primarily medium-chain fats.

- Goat cheese, sheep's milk cheese, butter, ghee, and similar dairy products contain primarily short and medium-chain fats in limited quantities.

- Starve chyle volume by limiting or avoiding:

- Other dairy foods, animal products, and meats that contain primarily long-chain fats.

- Oils and other fat-based ingredients in salad dressing and other foods.

- Fried foods and cooking fats (other than coconut oil) used in frying, baking, etc.

- Processed foods containing fats, especially chemically modified fats.

Leaky Lymphatics

Recent research shows enlarged and leaky lymphatic vessels (disrupted lymphatic vascular integrity) in mouse models of type 2 diabetes. Lymphatic leakage appears to be a general feature of diabetic lymphatic vasculature resulting in high blood pressure (hypertension), fat deposition, obesity, fibrosis, and inflammation. Lymphatic vessel function was rescued using L-arginine to increase nitric oxide availability [13].

L-arginine is the supplement form of arginine, a conditionally essential amino acid that supports many functions including regulating fat and protein metabolism. L-arginine supplements can be used to prevent and treat adiposity and metabolic syndrome [14].

Leakage from gut lymphatics contributes to intestinal edema, abdominal fat, abdominal swelling (abdominal panniculus), and edema of the trunk and lower extremities.

Food Choices and Leaky Lymphatics

Arginine is conditionally essential because healthy people synthesize adequate quantities internally and do not require any arginine from food sources. Dietary sources of arginine are needed when capacity for making arginine is reduced by conditions such as inflammation, infections, kidney problems or gut dysbiosis. Inflammation and disease-related conditions–especially liver disease (see "Fatty Liver Disease" on page 41)–increase levels of arginase, a competing enzyme that further reduces arginine and nitric oxide levels [15].

Eating to Starve Leaky Lymphatics

Fight leaky lymphatics by eating foods that help increase nitric oxide availability:

- Food sources of arginine such as fish, soy, beans, lentils, whole grains and nuts (including almonds and walnuts).

- Foods rich in nitrate/nitrite, the basis for nitric oxide: vegetables (especially green leafy vegetables) and fruits [16].

L-arginine supplements may be an appropriate first step towards better lymphatic vascular integrity if you have a condition that increases arginase levels, or if you are unable to increase nitric oxide levels by exercising regularly. This includes anyone with chronic venous insufficiency, congestive heart failure, type 2 diabetes, kidney disease, or liver disease. See "L-Arginine" on page 101.

Gut Microbes

Trillions of microbes) (bacteria, fungi, and viruses) live within our bodies (especially in the gut), on our skin, and on other body surfaces. We have a mutually beneficial relationship with this ecosystem. Gut microbes, in particular, provide many important functions.

Each person's community of microbes (microbiota) is unique and can be profiled based on the range of organism types (microbial diversity) and relative numbers of organisms of each type. Your microbiota has developed with you since birth (or earlier) and has been shaped by your experiences.

Factors that affect your microbiota include the genes you inherit (genetic factors), your birth process (vaginal delivery or cesarean section), people close to you, any pets, your environment, food choices, aging and life-cycle events (such as puberty, pregnancy, menopause, etc.), infections, diseases, surgery, antibiotics, medications, etc.

Microbiota Changes

Your personal microbiota profile is unique and remains stable over time. Some aspects of your gut microbiota are dynamic and change relatively quickly.

Changes take place on different time scales:

- Relative abundance of certain gut microbe types can change rapidly (within hours) in response to food, activity, or other factors. For example, a meal containing red meat triggers the release of bile acids, which leads to an increase in acid-loving gram-negative bacteria (such as E. coli), and a decrease in certain other types of bacteria.

- Diversity of gut microbes changes over somewhat longer periods based on habitual patterns. For example, frequently eating high-fat foods (multiple times per day for several days) increases the numbers of bile-loving microbes (such as pro-inflammatory B. wadsworthia), and the variety of specialized bile-loving bacteria types.

- Microbiota-induced changes in host gene expression are depend upon the specific genes involve, and the time required for these changes depends upon the turnover time of the host cells involved, and other factors.

Food choices are one of the major modulators of the intestinal microbiota and a dominant source of variation in its composition. Some aspects of your gut microbiota adapt within hours to changes in your eating pattern.

Antibiotics kill both helpful and harmful gut bacteria, thereby changing the balance between different varieties of bacteria and other microorganisms (such as yeast), reducing bacterial diversity, and contributing to an increase in antibiotic resistant types of bacteria. Antibiotic-related microbiota changes can result in weight gain, weight loss, or may not affect weight, depending on the type of antibiotic and your pre-treatment mix of microbes.

Other medications also affect gut microbes, especially medications where weight gain or weight loss is a common side effect. Gut microbiota changes from antibiotics and other medications happen within days and can be long lasting.

Stress, exercise, overall activity levels and timing of eating, fasting, and movement relative to the day-night cycle (diurnal cycle) also affect your microbiota. These changes are more subtle and take place over longer periods.

Gut Dysbiosis and Obesity

A healthy, or health promoting, microbiota (eubiosis) includes a diverse variety of microbe species and resists change under stress. Microbiota imbalance associated with disease (dysbiosis) has lower diversity, fewer beneficial microbes, more un-helpful bacteria and yeast (such as candida) and may include large quantities of disease-causing microbes (pathogens).

Animal studies have shown that obese and lean mice have different mixes of gut microbes. An obese mouse can be transformed into a lean mouse by transplanting the gut microbes from a lean mouse, and vice-versa [17].

Lymphedema and lipedema are associated with obesity promoting gut dysbiosis (obesogenic microbiota) characterized by increased numbers of acid-loving gram-negative bacteria and a reduction in beneficial, anti-inflammatory bacteria (such as Bifidobacterium and Lactobacillus). This includes overgrowth of a pathogenic type of E. coli (adherent-invasive type), resulting in increased intestinal permeability and inflammation, as well as significantly decreased levels of beneficial short-chain fatty acids.

Types of E. Coli

E. coli bacteria live in the intestines of humans and other animals. There are hundreds of different strains within the e. coli species, including many beneficial strains and a few pathological strains.

Beneficial strains include E. coli Nissle 1917, the only gram-negative bacteria used as a probiotic. This strain can help correct digestive disorders, including leaky gut (increased intestinal permeability).

Pathological strains of e. coli cause urinary tract infections, respiratory illness and pneumonia, and other illnesses. E. coli O157, the strain most commonly implicated in food-borne disease, lives in cows and similar animals. Illness can result from contaminated food or water, unpasteurized milk, contact with animals, or contact with the feces of infected people.

Although e. coli are only 0.1% of our gut bacteria, they play multiple roles in acquiring nutrients, preventing growth and colonization by bad bacteria, short-chain fatty acid production, and serotonin signaling. Serotonin signals influence local gut function, systemic metabolism, mood, and behavior. Our intestines contain multiple strains of e. coli and the mix of e. coli strains changes several times during the year as different strains displace each other.

This type of gut dysbiosis has wide-ranging effects on overall health and other medical conditions through obesity and related conditions. However, gut dysbiosis is not an infection or a gastrointestinal disorder, per se. If permitted to progress, gut dysbiosis may develop into a disorder such as celiac disease, irritable bowel syndrome (IBS), small intestine bacterial overgrowth (SIBO), etc.

Gut dysbiosis promotes weight gain by [18]:

- Harvesting more calories from food by slowing gut activity (low gut motility) and increasing absorption of sugars and fats.

- Low gut motility can also increase bile levels and gut-acidity by not allowing the gut to empty overnight and enter the fasting state, as explained below.

- Promoting fat storage and fat cell overgrowth.

- Interfering with the ability to use up (mobilize) stored fat as a source of energy.

- Increasing appetite and cravings for certain types of foods, especially carbohydrates and fats.

- Decreasing activity, energy expenditure, and mood.

Low gut motility can cause a variety of symptoms including bloating, pain after eating, altered bowel habits including constipation or diarrhea, etc. Certain foods may make symptoms worse such as greasy or rich foods, large quantities of foods with fiber, or beverages high in fat, sugar, or carbonation.

Gut dysbiosis contributes to other disease conditions including:

- Fatty liver disease by altering the metabolism of choline and bile acids, dysregulating alcohol elimination and, in a few people, fermenting carbohydrates into alcohol (endogenous alcohol production). See "Fatty Liver Disease" on page 41.

- Leaky lymphatic vessels by interfering with arginine synthesis and reducing nitric oxide availability. See "Leaky Lymphatics" on page 26.

- Systemic inflammation from endotoxins produced by gram-negative bacteria that enter the bloodstream via gut leakage triggered by the same bacteria, as explained below.

- Dysregulation of estrogen levels in the blood, as explained in "Maintaining Estrogen Regulation" on page 53.

- Congestive heart failure [19], chronic venous insufficiency [20], anxiety and depression.

Bile has an important role in creating the acidic environment that leads to this obesogenic dysbiosis and the over-growth of gram-negative bacteria. Bile acids produced by the liver are normally stored and concentrated in the gallbladder during the fasting state. Fasting between meals or overnight allows the intestine empty completely, become less acidic, and reduces the proportion of acid-loving bacteria. Extending the time between dinner and breakfast may help improve your health; see "Stay on Schedule" on page 202.

Fat entering the small intestine triggers endocrine cells to release cholecystokinin, a signaling hormone that causes multiple changes including:

- Stimulating the gallbladder to contract and release stored bile into the intestine. Bile makes the intestine more acidic and helps breakdown fats.

- Slowing gastric emptying and reducing gut motility.

- Increasing feelings of fullness (satiety) and decreasing appetite, in non-obese people. Signals to stop eating in response to high fat, high-energy foods appear to be impaired in obese people.

Several factors can disrupt the normal bile release cycle and maintain a more acidic environment in the small intestine, which allows gram-negative bacteria to proliferate:

- Liver disease impairs bile production and recirculation, resulting in an acidic environment. Many people with lymphedema or lipedema may also have liver disease; see "Fatty Liver Disease" on page 41.

- Endotoxins produced by gram-negative bacteria (discussed below) can trigger the release of bile by activating cells that produce cholecystokinin [21].

- Reduced gut motility caused by gram-negative bacteria, prolongs the time required to empty the gut and return to a normal intestinal acidity after eating, allowing the gut to remain acid for extended periods and promoting the growth of acid loving bacteria.

- Gall bladder removal surgery (cholecystectomy) results in a continuous flow of less concentrated bile into the small intestine, keeping the intestine acidic.

Food Choices and Gut Dysbiosis

Diets rich in saturated animal fats contribute to gut dysbiosis, and avoiding animal products or eating them infrequently and in limited quantities (5-8 servings per week) will help correct dysbiosis.

Kefir (a fermented milk product) may be helpful in reestablishing healthy gut bacteria because kefir has been shown to reverse the increase in gram-negative bacteria (B. wadsworthia) and increase the production of butyrate and other health-promoting short-chain fatty acids in the gut [22].

Gut Dysbiosis and Endotoxins

Systemic inflammation results when bacterial endotoxins from the small intestine are able to enter the blood circulation and activate the immune system. Chronic inflammation is characteristic of lymphedema and lipedema, as well as obesity, metabolic syndrome, diabetes, liver disease, etc.

Endotoxins, or lipopolysaccharides (LPS), are large molecules containing sugar and fat. These molecules come from the outer membrane of gram-negative bacteria and remain after the bacteria die. Contents of the small intestine include endotoxins from food-borne bacteria (killed by cooking) and gut bacteria. Gut dysbiosis increases the proportion of gram-negative bacteria in the gut, which increases endotoxin production.

Endotoxins gain entry into the blood via two pathways, both involving food choices and the lymphatic system):

- Fats from foods enable endotoxins to be absorbed into the intestinal villi lining the small intestine along with other components of chyle, which then flows through the lacteals, into the central lymphatic vessels, and bloodstream, as described above.

- Gut leakage (increased intestinal permeability) caused by gluten, gram-negative bacteria, or other triggers allows endotoxins (and other gut contents) to enter the wall of the small intestine and be collected by the lymphatic system and passed into the blood (see "Gut Leakage" on page 37).

Food Choices and Endotoxins

Food choices can increase endotoxin production in the gut and the ability of endotoxins to enter the bloodstream.

Endotoxins are produced from sugar and fat. These ingredients can come from the same food (such as cream containing milk sugar or lactose and milk fat) or food combinations (such as a fast-food breakfast with bread, egg, cheese, fried potatoes, etc.). Sugars can be from any carbohydrate including grain-based foods that are rapidly converted to glucose.

Foods containing long-chain fats facilitate endotoxin entry into the blood circulation via chyle. Gluten containing foods (wheat, rye, barley) can increase gut leakage and permit endotoxin entry via that pathway, as discussed below.

Fats (especially milk fat) and possibly fructose have the greatest potential for increasing endotoxins and inflammation. Mice given high-fructose drinks had a 27-fold increase in endotoxin levels [23].

Milk fat in highly concentrated form (anhydrous milk fat) is used abundantly in processed and confectionary foods, and occurs naturally in cream, milk, and other dairy products. Normal-weight study participants who drank a small serving of cream (33 g. or about 1 oz.) had a significant increase in endotoxin levels and endotoxin levels were still increasing five hours later [24]. Mice fed milk fat developed inflammation, colitis, and overgrowth of certain bacteria but mice in the same study fed other types of fat (lard, safflower oil) did not develop inflammation [25].

In a different study, mice raised on cream from grass-fed cows developed less fat and inflammation, despite a higher food intake, than mice fed standard dairy cream. These differences were attributed to the greater omega-3 fat content of the grass-fed cream [26].

Combinations of foods have different inflammatory results. Adding other foods can reduce the pro-inflammatory effects of a high-fat and high-carb meal. For example orange juice containing anti-inflammatory flavonoids muted the inflammatory effects of a fast-food breakfast [27].

Eating to Starve Gut Dysbiosis

Feed health-promoting microbes:

- Fermented foods, especially kefir, a fermented milk product containing helpful bacteria (see "Fermented Foods" on page 90).

- Colorful vegetables (especially cruciferous vegetables) and fruits, the more varieties the better. Green leafy vegetables contain unique nutrients (such as sulfoquinovose) that promote growth of protective strains of E. coli.

- Citrus and other foods containing anti-inflammatory flavonoids.

- Dietary fiber, especially inulin fiber from food sources or supplements (see "Inulin" on page 87).

- Omega-3 fats from fatty fish, grass-fed diary, etc. See "Omega-3 vs. Omega-6 Fats" on page 85.

- Spices and herbs that fight inflammation such as cinnamon, cloves, ginger, rosemary, turmeric, etc.

Starve (or do not promote) un-helpful microbes by limiting or avoiding:

- Fats in general, especially animal fats from dairy products containing fat and sugars (cream, milk, ice cream, etc.) and meats.

- Meals combining fats with carbohydrates from simple sugars or grain-based foods, especially grains containing gluten.

- Fructose in sugar-sweetened beverages, fruit drinks, high fructose sweeteners, etc.

- Processed foods and fast food made with anhydrous milk fat.

Probiotics and calcium-D-glucarate supplements (see "Calcium-D-Glucarate" on page 104) can help reestablish healthy gut bacteria, if needed [28].

Grain and Gluten Metabolism

Grains are seeds from grass-like plants that must be processed before use in food to remove the tough outer covering. Most grains are ground into flour before cooking. Grains are a major part of the Western diet; many Americans get more than half their calories from wheat. Most processed foods are grain-based, or include grain-based additives.

Grains of all types raise glucose levels quickly, which has a number of implications for health, and affects everyone, as explained below.

Gluten is a mixture of proteins that provides the 'glue' to make dough elastic and bread chewy. Gluten occurs naturally in the seeds of wheat, rye, barley, and certain other grains.

Many people are unable to fully digest gluten and react in ways that affect their health, even without clearly identifiable symptoms. Reactions vary based on number of factors including genetics, autoimmune disorders, gut microbiota composition, etc. Gluten or wheat can cause a number of different reactions. We only describe the conditions that likely to increase edema: gut leakage, non-celiac gluten sensitivity, and celiac disease.

In some people who are sensitive to gluten, eating gluten appears to cause the same type of obesogenic gut dysbiosis discussed above with an overgrowth of E. coli and other gram-negative bacteria. Gut dysbiosis caused by gluten sensitivity can be reversed by a gluten-free diet [29].

Grains and Glucose Levels

Grains contain a mix of nutrients but are primarily complex carbohydrates or starches. Starches from grain-based foods are quickly converted into sugar or glucose by microbes in the small intestine, resulting in a rapid increase in glucose availability. White bread and certain other grain-based products raise blood glucose levels more quickly than table sugar.

Effects of rapidly increased glucose availability in the gut include:

- Glucose absorption into the blood: raising blood glucose levels rapidly, which signals the pancreas to release insulin. Everyone experiences this increase but the increase in glucose levels is not apparent in non-diabetics because their bodies compensate automatically by releasing more insulin.

- Inflammatory endotoxin production: if fats are present, gram-negative gut bacteria form endotoxins, bacterial fragments combining sugar and fat, as discussed above.

- Fat accumulation in the liver: sugar is converted into fat and stored under conditions where both glucose and insulin levels are high. Elevated glucose levels contribute to fatty liver disease, see "Fatty Liver Disease" on page 41.

- Sharp decrease in blood glucose levels (hypoglycemia): high glucose and insulin levels cause blood glucose to drop several hours later, triggering hunger and increased food intake, which contributes to obesity.

Patient Experience

I have almost eliminated wheat from my diet and it is now an occasional treat. Over the past year, I have noticed that my digestion has improved and the areas of lymphedema that I battle, although they have never been severe, have now become nearly unnoticeable. Particularly, the lymphedema that I tend to fight in my lateral trunk has become a very rare irritant and it used to bother me daily. I'm quite pleased with the results I have had from changing my diet, and it was not really very difficult to do.
AMK

- Metabolic syndrome and diabetes due to loss of the insulin-secreting function of the pancreatic beta cells as a result of frequent high blood glucose levels and excessive insulin secretion.

- Increased risk for cardiovascular disease and other health conditions.

Eating to Starve Grains and Glucose Levels

Starve elevated glucose levels by minimizing:

- Grain-based foods of all types, especially those made with grains containing gluten (wheat, rye and barley) or flour (refined grains).

- Processed or manufactured foods containing refined grain-based ingredients or additives.

- Gluten-free (or more properly gluten-substitute) breads, pizza, baked goods, etc. In place of wheat, these use other starches that raise glucose quickly such as rice flour, potato starch, tapioca, etc.

Oats do not contain gluten but may be contaminated by wheat during processing. For a strictly gluten-free diet look for oats labelled gluten free.

Gut Leakage

Cells lining the interior of the small intestine are connected by tight junctions, a barrier mechanism that can open and close. Opening these junctions allows large molecules to enter wall of the small intestine (the submucosa).

This barrier plays an important role in immune system surveillance and protection.

Tight junction barrier functions are controlled by zonulin, a signaling protein. Elevated zonulin levels cause gut leakage (increased intestinal permeability) by opening the tight junctions. Elevated zonulin levels and increased intestinal permeability are characteristics of certain autoimmune disorders (celiac disease, type 1 diabetes, etc.) and other conditions.

Gut leakage allows large molecules to enter the blood stream and trigger systemic inflammation. Molecules that gain entry via this mechanism include:

- Endotoxins from gram-negative bacteria, as discussed above.

- Gluten and other proteins, peptides, and lectins from wheat, rye or barley.

About 40% of the population has genes for gluten sensitivity (HLA-DQ2 or HLA-DQ8) and may react to leaked gluten components that enter the blood stream and trigger the adaptive immune system. Gluten sensitivity and dietary gluten can lead to edema, gastrointestinal symptoms including weight gain or loss, diabetes, rheumatoid arthritis, neurological impairment, and other health issues.

Zonulin release and gut leakage can be triggered by several stimuli. Two of the most powerful triggers are:

- Gram-negative bacteria overgrowth from enteric infection or gut dysbiosis.

- Gluten (specifically the gliadin protein) from foods containing wheat, rye, or barley. Gluten-related gut leakage has an important role in non-celiac gluten sensitivity and celiac disease (discussed below), but is not limited to persons with genetic factors for these conditions.

Gut permeability and zonulin levels can be reduced by certain foods; for example, citrus fruits containing flavonoids.

Eating to Starve Gut Leakage

Starve gut leakage by:

- Eating to starve gut dysbiosis as explained above.

- Avoiding foods containing gluten from wheat, rye, or barley, as well as gluten-based meat substitutes.

Non-Celiac Gluten Sensitivity

Non-Celiac Gluten Sensitivity (NCGS) affects about 10% of the population. NCGS symptoms include many that are common in people with lymphedema–fatigue, joint and muscle pain, leg or arm numbness, and depression–as well as dermatitis, anemia, abdominal pain, bloating, diarrhea or constipation. In NCGS these symptoms occur soon after eating gluten, disappear with gluten withdrawal, and reappear within hours or days after gluten is reintroduced [30].

Although gluten increases NCGS symptoms, fructans and other fermentable carbohydrates (FODMAP foods) trigger NCGS and irritable bowel syndrome (IBS) [31]. FODMAP compounds are found in wheat and rye, as well as certain vegetables, fruits, beans, and inulin fiber supplements.

Eating to Starve Non-Celiac Gluten Sensitivity

Non-celiac gluten sensitivity is a condition where your mileage may vary, depending on your specific triggers, your degree of sensitivity to these triggers, and combinations of foods. Keeping a Food Diary may help you identify your triggers (see "Food Diary" on page 226).

Starve non-celiac gluten sensitivity by:

- Avoiding foods made with gluten-containing grains: wheat, rye, and barley; as well as gluten-based meat substitutes.

- Minimizing foods containing FODMAP carbohydrates, as necessary. FODMAP foods are indicated in the shopping guide (Appendix A).

Celiac Disease

Gluten sensitivity, gluten in the diet, and some as yet unknown environmental factors (such as an infection) results in celiac disease, an autoimmune disorder where gluten activates both the innate and adaptive immune systems in the small intestine.

Symptoms of celiac disease vary widely and can overlap with other disorders. Some people with celiac disease develop cramps and diarrhea from even a single crumb of bread.

Celiac disease appears to be increasingly common, especially in people over 60 years of age who often have vitamin and mineral deficiencies without GI symptoms. Untreated celiac disease can cause anemia, calcium and vitamin D deficiencies, osteoporosis, osteomalacia, lactose intolerance, and increased cancer risk [32].

Celiac disease is under-diagnosed because many people do not have gastrointestinal symptoms [33]. Risk factors for celiac disease include Turner syndrome (a form of primary lymphedema), family members with celiac disease or gluten sensitivity, autoimmune thyroid disease, type 1 diabetes, and other autoimmune diseases [34].

One sign of celiac disease is damage to the villi lining the small intestine. As described above, villi contain lymphatic capillaries that convey partially digested fats into the lymphatic system. Intestinal lymphatic damage from celiac disease or other causes can result in edema or lymphedema of the trunk and legs. Chyle leakage (chylous ascites) or excess fluid in the lining of the lungs (pleural effusion) may occur in severe cases [35].

Gluten is established as the instigator of autoimmunity in celiac disease and this autoimmune process is halted by removing gluten from the diet. A strict gluten-free diet allows the damaged intestinal villi to heal and may reverse many celiac symptoms within 6 to 24 months, for most people [36]. People also report better overall health and energy.

Eating to Starve Celiac Disease

See the resource list in Appendix E for more information on diet for celiac disease.

Starve celiac disease by following a strict gluten-free diet:

- No foods containing wheat, rye, or barley; no gluten-based meat substitutes.

- Avoid oats and other grains that may be cross contaminated by gluten unless they are labeled as gluten free.

- Check labels for hidden sources of gluten such as wheat-based soy sauce, food starch, and certain food additives (see the ingredient list in Appendix B).

Limit or avoid gluten-free (or more properly gluten-substitute) breads, pizza, baked goods, etc. In place of wheat, these use other starches that raise glucose quickly such as rice flour, potato starch, tapioca, etc.

Liver

The liver provides a wide variety of functions to support and regulate the metabolism. This section focuses on the liver as a major source of lymph under normal conditions and greatly increased lymph volumes if the liver is diseased.

Other relevant aspects of the liver include:

- The role of the liver in creating bile, as mentioned in the discussion of gut dysbiosis above.

- The role of the liver in regulating estrogen levels is covered in "Maintaining Estrogen Regulation" on page 53.

Fatty Liver Disease

Obesity and metabolic syndrome result in fat accumulation and tissue changes that reduces liver function in children, adolescents, and adults. Nonalcoholic fatty liver disease (NAFLD) is the most common chronic liver disease in the US.

NAFLD starts with abnormal fat production and build-up in the liver (hepatic steatosis) and can progress to a stage of inflammation and liver damage known as nonalcoholic steatohepatitis (NASH), followed by life-threatening cirrhosis or liver cancer.

NAFLD cannot be diagnosed without biopsy or imaging and frequently has no symptoms in the early stages. When symptoms occur, they may include swelling of the legs (edema) and abdomen (ascites), fatigue, weakness, weight loss, loss of appetite, nausea, abdominal pain, spider-like blood vessels, yellowing of the skin and eyes (jaundice), itching, and mental confusion.

Risk of NAFLD increases with weight. In American adults, NAFLD affects 15% of non-obese adults, 65% of adults with a BMI of 30-40, and 85% of adults with a BMI above 40 [37]. In North American children and adolescents (age 1-19), NAFLD affects 7% of the general population and 39% of those who are obese (BMI >25) [38].

A healthy liver creates about half the total lymph volume in the body. NAFLD increases lymph production by the liver at each stage of the disease, as abnormal fat accumulates and liver function decreases. In late-stage NAFLD or cirrhosis, the damaged liver produces 6 to 10 times the normal lymph volume and increased lymph flow can stretch the thoracic duct to 2 to 4 times its normal diameter. Increased pressure can cause lymph to weep from the surface of the liver and accumulate in the abdomen (ascites) or lungs (pleural effusion) [39].

Increased lymph volume from liver disease, combined with leaky lymphatic vessels (increased lymphatic permeability), contributes to intestinal edema, abdominal fat, abdominal swelling (abdominal panniculus), and edema of the trunk, genitals, and lower extremities.

Gut microbes play an important role in liver health. Gut dysbiosis, gut leakage (increased gut permeability) and inflammation from endotoxins are common in people with NAFLD, as is small intestine bacterial overgrowth (SIBO). Prebiotics such as inulin fiber (see "Inulin" on page 87) and probiotics show promise as NAFLD treatments but larger studies are needed [40].

Food Choices and Fatty Liver Disease

Carbohydrates containing glucose and fructose–especially concentrated forms of fructose used in drinks and packaged foods–can induce NAFLD by increasing fat creation in the liver (de novo lipogenesis) and promoting liver fibrosis. High-fructose corn syrup (HFCS) contains 55 to 90% fructose, agave nectar is 70 to 90% fructose, honey is about 70% fructose, sugar (sucrose) is 50% fructose and 50% glucose, and high-fructose fruits such as grapes or apples are 5-10% fructose [41].

Pear, apple, and other fruit concentrates used to sweeten drinks and processed foods are also high in fructose. Popular beverages made with HFCS contain 50% more fructose than glucose while some 'pure fruit juices' have twice as much fructose as glucose [42].

Ninety-eight percent of postmenopausal American women risk liver damage by not getting adequate choline–given that women need more choline from food sources as estrogen levels decline during menopause. Choline deficiency causes muscle damage as well as abnormal fat deposition in the liver. Recommended choline intake is at least 425 mg/day for women and 550 mg/day for men [43].

Eating to Starve Fatty Liver Disease

Eat foods that support healthy liver function including:

- Cruciferous vegetables, whole eggs. seafood and other foods rich in choline.

- Fatty fish, dark green leafy vegetables, and other sources of unsaturated fats that help reduce fat storage in the liver, especially omega-3 and omega-6 fats (see "Omega-3 vs. Omega-6 Fats" on page 85), as well as monosaturated fats from plant sources like olive oil, nuts, and avocados [44].

- Food containing inulin or inulin supplements (see "Inulin Fiber" on page 100).

Starve liver disease by limiting or avoiding these foods:

- Sugar and fructose in sugar sweetened beverages, fruit juices, sweets, processed foods, high-fructose sweeteners, etc. Limit fruits that are high in fructose, such as apples and pears.

- Refined grains and other carbohydrates that raise blood glucose levels quickly and trigger the release of insulin, signaling the liver to convert glucose into stored fat.

- Alcohol, which can cause or increase liver inflammation and promotes fat storage in the liver.

- Saturated fats from meats or dairy foods because excess fat contributes to fat accumulation in the liver.

Balancing calorie intake and energy usage to avoid over nutrition is important for avoiding or correcting NAFLD.

Skin

Skin, our largest and most exposed organ, provides a barrier to the external environment that can resist a wide range of challenges. The skin, and the lymphatics within the skin, also play important roles in regulating blood pressure, fluid balance, sodium levels, and body temperature. Injury or infection increase the amount of tissue fluid in the affected area.

Lymphatic collectors and the initial lymphatic vessels are very tiny tubes located just below the surface of the skin. Skin movements open tiny button junctions in the walls of the lymphatic collectors, allowing tissue fluid to flow into the lymphatic system. These delicate little vessels are easily damaged will not function if compressed by external pressure, or if the larger lymphatic vessels they drain into are overloaded with fluid.

Excess fluid or chyle can flow backwards into the skin if the lymphatic system is overloaded. Under these conditions, lymphatic collectors leak and lymph or chyle escapes through the skin, a condition known as weeping lymphedema (lymphorrhea).

In the early stages of lymphedema the affected tissues remain soft, and swollen areas will indent if pressed (pitting edema). Swelling may stretch the skin, causing pain, and damaging the nerves.

Skin affected by lymphedema is vulnerable to infection (cellulitis) from common skin bacteria (streptococcus or staphylococcus). If bacteria are able to penetrate the skin, they grow rapidly in the protein-rich tissue fluid trapped within the skin.

Lymph flow and lymph processing within the lymph nodes are important mechanisms for detecting and fighting infections, as well as healing damaged tissues. Immune system functions are impaired in areas affected by lymphedema (or at risk for lymphedema), especially where lymph nodes have been removed or damaged. Wounds or ulcers in affected areas may not heal for similar reasons.

As lymphedema progresses to later stages, stagnant tissue fluid (lymph stasis) causes abnormal tissue fiber growth (fibrosis) and fat accumulation, resulting in hard tissue that will not indent when pressed (non-pitting edema).

Without effective treatment, fat will continue to accumulate in affected areas. Fat deposits on the affected limbs or the abdomen (abdominal panniculus) can become disfiguring. The weight of accumulated fat, abnormal posture or gait, and joint damage from excess fluid can cause disabling orthopedic problems.

Acid Barrier

The acid barrier, or acid mantle, is a thin layer of sweat and oils secreted by the sebaceous glands that protects the skin by limiting the growth of surface bacteria and preventing bacteria from entering the skin. Skin becomes thinner with aging and lymphedema, and the acid barrier may weaken. Alkaline or basic chemicals, cleaners, soaps, detergents, shampoos, peels, hair removers, or skin care products damage the acid barrier and should be avoided.

Salt and Skin

Recent findings show high salt intake results in salt being stored in the skin as sodium and chloride ions. Immune cells regulate this storage, along with blood pressure and other lymphatic functions. Immune system Mononuclear Phagocyte System cells (MPS cells) sense sodium levels and respond with biological signals including VEGF to modify the volume of lymph, the balance between water and electrolytes (including sodium) in the tissue fluid, and blood pressure. Over time, a high salt diet results in abnormal lymphatic capillary growth (hyperplasia) in the skin [45] and reduces lymphatic pumping activity [46].

A high salt diet also increases the number of Th17 cells (Interleukin-17 producing CD4+ helper T cells) that are highly stable, pathogenic, and pro-inflammatory. Th17 cells are associated with increased risk of developing several autoimmune disorders including psoriasis, rheumatoid arthritis, and asthma [47].

Food Choices and Skin

Food choices influence lymphedema-related skin changes through several mechanisms including:

- Colorful vegetables and fruits including dark green leafy vegetables provide many nutrients that support skin health and fight diseases.

- Omega-3 fats in adequate quantities to support the acid barrier while limiting pro-inflammatory omega-6 fats (see "Omega-3 vs. Omega-6 Fats" on page 85).

- Salt intake within the recommended range so that sodium levels are neither too low nor too high. See "Sodium" on page 79.

Foods choices also affect the skin via other relationships discussed in this chapter:

- Liver disease contributes to skin edema by increasing the amount of lymph produced by the liver, raising the pressure in the central lymphatic vessels, and interfering with lymph drainage from the skin.

- Increased chyle volume also increases pressure in the central lymphatic vessels and contributes to edema.

- Circulating endotoxins cause inflammation, edema, and cell damage in the skin.

- Biological signals contribute to skin damage in several ways including abnormal Vascular Endothelial Growth Factor (VEGF) signals that cause overgrowth of dysfunctional lymphatic vessels and abnormal Fibrosis Growth Factor 2 (FGF2) signals that cause the overgrowth of skin tissue fibers (fibrosis).

Restricting fluid intake or dietary protein will *not* reduce the risk of skin infections and can make swelling worse. Diuretics are not recommended treatment for lymphedema because they can increase the risk of tissue hardening (fibrosis) by concentrating tissue fluid.

Abnormal Biological Signals

Biological signals coordinate bodily processes through a balance of pro- and anti-signaling factors. Important signaling factors related to lymphedema include VEGF which regulates blood and lymphatic vessel growth and FGF2 which promotes tissue hardening (fibrosis).

People with, or at risk for, lymphedema and lipedema have multiple sources of abnormal VEGF and FGF2 signals:

- Primary lymphedema is caused by genetic defects that affect VEGF signaling and result in missing lymphatic structures, smaller than normal lymph vessels, overgrowth of vessels, and/or ineffective lymph vessels [48]. VEGF levels are higher in patients with primary lymphedema than in healthy controls [49]. High VEGF levels in primary lymphedema also cause abnormal and leaky blood vessels, resulting in tissue edema [50].

- Tumors use biological signals, including VEGF and FGF2, to trigger:

  - Abnormal blood vessel growth to create a blood supply to tumors. Tumors cannot grow beyond the size of a pinhead without their own blood supply [51].

  - Growth of abnormal lymphatic vessels that enable cancer to spread (metastasize) to draining lymph nodes and distant organs via the lymphatic system and inhibit the normal immune system response.

  - Fibrosis of the skin, which also inhibits immune system response.

  - Lymphedema and decreased immune system response. This helps explain why 15% of breast cancer patients had impaired lymphatic drainage *before treatment or lymph node removal* [52].

- Lipedema patients had plasma VEGF levels nearly four times higher than controls without lipedema [53].

- Acute inflammation triggers VEGF to promote lymph vessel growth and clear infection and inflammation. Chronic inflammation also triggers lymphatic vessel growth via VEGF but the resulting abnormal lymphatic vessels are not functional and increase swelling [54].

Adipose tissues create more fat by releasing biological signals that increase appetite and food intake, insulin resistance, chronic inflammation, and the rate of fat storage [55]. Macrophages in adipose tissue secrete signaling factors including VEGF which trigger the formation of leaky lymphatic vessels leading to further swelling, inflammation, and obesity [56].

Stress of several types triggers biological signals including VEGF. These stresses include [57]:

- Low tissue oxygen levels (hypoxia) caused by high blood pressure (hypertension), diabetes, Alzheimer's disease, asthma and other respiratory conditions, smoking, high altitudes, air travel, etc.

- Mechanical stress from tight garments, belts, straps, jewelry, shoes, etc. or pressure from body weight or other body parts. Gentle pressure from properly fitted compression garments does not trigger stress signals.

- Metabolic stress such as low blood sugar (hypoglycemia), high blood sugar (hyperglycemia), or gut dysbiosis (overgrowth of gram-negative bacteria).

- Psychosocial stress such as disabling work stress, stressful family relationships, or a combination of stressors [58].

Cigarette smoke interferes with normal VEGF signaling—in addition to stressing cells—and should be avoided by anyone with, or at risk for, lymphedema [59].

Food Choices and Abnormal Biological Signals

Certain foods we recommend—primarily colorful vegetables and fruits—fight abnormal biological signals and inflammation. Many of these foods also offer other health benefits.

Colors in plants signal the presence of different types of nutrients. For example, red from lycopene in tomatoes, and black or purple color from anthocyanins in berries or grapes. Eating plants with many colors (rainbow-colored) provides a range of different nutrients and eating more varieties of vegetables increases gut microbe diversity.

Table 2-1: Food Sources of Anti-Angiogenic Factors

Food Sources	Anti-angiogenic Factors	Blocks VEGF or FGF2
Green Tea	Green Tea Catechins	Yes
Soybeans	Genistein	Yes
Mulberries, peanuts, grapes, and grape products, including red and rosé wine	Resveratrol	Yes
Tomatoes, watermelon, papaya, other bright red fruits	Lycopene	Yes
Cold water oily fish, flaxseed, nuts, etc.	Omega-3 fats	
Cruciferous vegetables including cabbage, broccoli, cauliflower, collard greens, mustard greens, radishes, Brussels sprouts, bok choy, and kale	Glucosinolates, Isothiocyanates, and Indole-3-carbinol	
Spinach, onions, parsley, beets, and thyme	Flavonoids	Yes
Salad greens such as lettuce, chicory, arugula, and red lettuce	Polyphenolic flavonoids	Yes
Berries, grapes, and red wine	Anthocyanidins	Yes
Cacao (source of chocolate), cinnamon, cranberry, apples, grapes, black currants, chokeberry, and persimmon	Proanthocyanidins	Yes
Fruits and nuts including pomegranate, strawberries, blackberries, raspberries, muscadine grapes, walnuts, and pecans	Ellagitannins	Yes
Cheese, yogurt, fermented soy (such as natto), and dark meat	Menaquinone (vitamin K2)	
Turmeric	Curcumin	Yes
Bright orange, red, or yellow foods	Beta-cryptoxanthin	

Research looking at way to fight cancer by cutting off the blood supply to tumors resulted in drugs that combat abnormal blood vessel growth. Anti-angiogenic drugs inhibit the biological signals promoting abnormal growth. Avastin (bevacizumab) for example, blocks abnormal VEGF signals promoting the growth of blood and lymph vessels [60].

Additional research identified chemical factors in vegetables, fruits, and other foods capable of counteracting VEGF and other abnormal biological signals from tumors or other sources. Certain foods are as effective as drugs in blocking abnormal vessel growth.

Tests of 34 types of vegetables against 8 types of tumor cells showed that dark green, cruciferous vegetables, onions and garlic (allium family) showed potent anti-cancer and anti-inflammatory properties. The most common vegetables in Western diets (potato, carrot, lettuce, and tomato) had little effect [61].

Eating to Starve Abnormal Biological Signals

Eat 'fighting foods' to counteract abnormal biological signals including colorful vegetables and fruits and other foods, that contain naturally occurring compounds shown to counter abnormal biological signals and their negative effects.

"Table 2-1: Food Sources of Anti-Angiogenic Factors" on page 49 shows foods that are sources of anti-angiogenic factors based on William Li's paper on dietary cancer prevention [62]. Many of these factors block abnormal VEGF or FGF2 signaling (as shown in the right column), and fight inflammation.

Lipedema Fat

Lipedema fat has a number of unique characteristics. Leaks in tiny blood and lymph vessels (microaneurysms) are characteristic features of lipedema fat and one of the earliest signs of the condition. Leakage may be due to genetic abnormalities in VEGF signaling that makes new vessels leaky and immature [63].

Lipedema fat cells differ metabolically from normal fat. Fat cells in affected areas become very large, another marker of affected fat tissue. Cells undergo accelerated cycles of cell death and simultaneous regeneration, recruiting immune cells, and resulting in chronically inflamed tissues. Compared to normal fat, lipedema tissues have many more crown-like-structures formed by macrophages scavenging debris from dying fat cells and stem/progenitor/stromal cells for growing and repairing fat cells [64].

Nerve damage and pain in areas affected by lipedema result from impaired circulation, lack of adequate blood supply for enlarged fat cells, mechanical forces from edema and fat expansion, and inflammation. Immobility or reduced ability to perceive movement due to nerve damage contribute to fat accumulation [65]. Nerve damage and lack of movement also contribute to fat proliferation in areas affected by lymphedema. SLD, MLD, exercise, and compression can help counter this effect.

Fat (adipose tissue) acts as an endocrine organ and secretes a number of signaling proteins for metabolic regulation including leptin and adiponectin. Leptin stimulates energy expenditure and inhibits food intake but obesity related gut dysbiosis reduces its effects. Adiponectin increases insulin sensitivity, fatty acid oxidation, and energy expenditure while reducing glucose production by the liver but obesity reduces adiponectin secretion.

Lipedema fat cells take in glucose and convert it to stored fat when insulin and glucose levels are high. Elevated insulin and glucose levels are characteristics of insulin resistance and type 2 diabetes. Macrophage activity and inflammation, as well as menopause and other hormone changes that increase lipedema fat, are linked to insulin resistance. Abnormal fat growth in lipedema appears to be particularly sensitive to excess glucose and insulin, possibly enhanced by an inherited variation in how estrogen-related hormones influence fat cell growth.

Lipedema Fat and Estrogens

Estrogens are a concern for both lipedema and lymphedema because they promote fat expansion as well as breast cancer, cancers of the reproductive tract, and other reproductive disorders. Estrogens are also important regulators of skin health, metabolism, electrolyte balance, and the cardiovascular system.

Pre-menopausal women synthesize estrogen from cholesterol in the ovaries and other organs. Women of all ages and men synthesize estrogen from testosterone, androstenedione, dehydroepiandrosterone (DHEA) and dehydroepiandrosterone sulfate (DHEAS) in fat and other tissues that are not part of the reproductive system (extragonadal estrogen) [66]. Estrogen from fat cells can act locally within the fat cell, affect nearby cells, or enter the blood stream and affect other parts of the body.

Many types of estrogens and estrogen-like compounds are found in animal and plant based foods. During the digestive process, gut microbes convert these compounds into a mix of different estrogen metabolites. Estrogen metabolites vary in terms of their effects on overall health and their other properties.

Estrogen and estrogen-like compounds circulating in the blood can bind to specialized receptors (estrogen receptors) in many parts of the body. Levels of estrogen compounds circulating in the blood are controlled by gut bacteria and the liver, as explained below.

Estrogen, together with genetic factors, appears to drive lipedema fat growth through multiple mechanisms including [67]:

- Increasing body region-specific fat accumulation on the hips and legs.

- Blocking fat cell mobilization that could deplete fat stores on the hips and legs.

- Increasing appetite and interfering with food intake versus energy expenditure regulation by the hypothalamus and sympathetic nervous system via leptin, insulin, ghrelin, and other biological signals.

Estrogen-controlled fat distribution results in increased fat on the buttocks and thighs (gluteal-femoral region), rather than the abdominal region. Estrogen appears to preserve fat on the buttocks and thighs (by suppressing fat mobilization)—but not the abdomen—in response to exercise or other energy demands [68].

In women, lipedema fat develops almost exclusively during times when estrogen levels are high: during puberty, pregnancy, and around the menopause transition Estrogen levels rise steeply before declining into menopause in some women [69].

Difference in estrogen levels by race/ethnicity are consistent with patterns observed in women seeking care for lipedema. Asian women rarely develop lipedema. Chinese and Japanese women in the US have generally lower estrogen levels overall and their estrogen levels follow a low-concentration decline trajectory, without an increase prior to declining into menopause [70].

Men with lipedema are rare and frequently have abnormal hormone levels due to deficiencies (testosterone or growth hormone) or liver disease.

Lipedema pain may be increased by certain estrogen metabolites (estradiol-3-glucuronide and estradiol-17-glucuronide) that enhance pain by activating specific pattern recognition receptors in the central nervous system (toll-like receptor 4) [71].

Food Choices and Lipedema Fat/Estrogen

Food choices to help minimize lipedema fat by normalizing estrogen levels include:

- Maintaining normal blood estrogen levels and health promoting gut microbes capable of regulating blood estrogen levels (as explained below) by correcting gut dysbiosis (as discussed above).

- Minimizing dietary estrogens and cholesterol from meats and animal products.

- Moderating intake of plant-based estrogens from soy.

- Adding lignans to your eating pattern.

- Influencing estrogen metabolism to favor beneficial metabolites.

Some people with lipedema are so sensitive to salt that one pickle can trigger a major weight increase. It is not clear if, or how, lymphedema affects salt-related weight changes but limiting salt is important.

Maintaining Estrogen Regulation

The amount of estrogen circulating in the blood is regulated by the estrobolome, a collection of gastrointestinal bacteria in the small intestine. Gut dysbiosis (discussed above) interferes with estrogen regulation, which leads to abnormal estrogen levels. Correcting or avoiding gut dysbiosis should maintain estrogen regulation capability and keep estrogens within a healthy range.

Certain estrogen compounds (conjugated estrogens) are removed from the blood by the liver and passed into the small intestine via bile. Depending on the mix of bacteria in the intestine, conjugated estrogens can either be deconjugated and returned to the blood stream (enterohepatic circulation) or converted into estrogen compounds that will be excreted via urine or feces. Changing the mix of estrobolome bacteria results in estrogen dysregulation and either abnormally high or low levels of circulating estrogens [72].

Elevated estrogen levels can result from diets rich in fats or red meat, which increase production of bile acids for fat digestion. Bacteria break down the bile acids into metabolites that promote the growth of E. coli and other gram-negative bacteria while reducing the numbers of beneficial Firmicutes and Bacteroidetes bacteria. E. coli produce enzymes that deconjugate estrogens and allow estrogens to return to the blood stream, increasing estrogen levels and potency. This microbial imbalance (dysbiosis) and overgrowth of gram-negative bacteria also promotes obesity (obesogenic gut microbes). Related gut bacteria changes reduce the body's ability to fight inflammation, infection, and cancer by removing killer T cells and lymphocytes [73].

Minimize Estrogen and Cholesterol from Animal Products

Not eating meat (vegan or vegetarian eating pattern) or eating less meat has been shown to lower estrogen levels in pre-menopausal women [74]. Estrogen may be lower because of less dietary cholesterol from animal products (cholesterol is converted to estrogen), less estrogen and phytoestrogen from meats, or better estrogen regulation (animal fats disrupt estrogen regulation by gut microbes as discussed above).

In the US, most cattle receive estrogen implants to promote rapid weight gain. American beef contains higher levels of estrogen in the meat, especially estrogens of the type contained in the implants, compared to Japanese beef raised without supplemental hormones [75].

Moderate Plant-Based Estrogens from Soy

Plant-based estrogens or phytoestrogens are naturally occurring plant compounds with chemical structures similar enough to estrogen that they can bind to estrogen receptors in the body. Estrogen binding capability also makes phytoestrogens potential endocrine-disrupting chemicals capable of interfering with normal hormonal and reproductive system functions.

Phytoestrogens are abundant in certain plants, especially soybeans and other legumes. Dietary sources of phytoestrogens also include meat and animal products from animals raised on feeds containing soy or other plant sources of phytoestrogens.

Dietary soy effects levels of estrogen and other sex hormones but these changes vary based on the type and quantity of soy, genetic or ethnic factors related to phytoestrogen metabolism, gut microbiota, and possibly other dietary or environmental factors. Some studies show soy lowers serum estrogen levels while other studies showed soy reduces estrogen elimination (urinary estrogens and metabolites) [76].

Only 30% of the western population have the ability to benefit from soy by converting soy protein into equol, an antioxidant and health-promoting metabolite, instead of the obesity promoting alternative (O-desmethylangolensin). Asian populations, 60% of which are equol producers, have a lower incidence of hormone-dependent diseases while consuming a soy-based diet [77].

Fermented organic soy foods are more beneficial than non-fermented soy because fermentation increases availability of phytoestrogens by breaking down soy proteins and as well as providing anti-angiogenic menaquinone (vitamin K2) and beneficial bacteria.

See if these soy foods work for you:

- Organic soybeans or edamame.

- Organic tofu.

- Fermented soy: miso, natto, soy-only soy sauce (shoyu), tempeh, tofu that is fermented or pickled (regular tofu is not fermented).

Moderate intake of soy-based estrogens by avoiding foods containing processed unfermented soy:

- Soy-based foods: soymilk, soy-based infant formula, and soy-based nutritional supplements.

- Meat substitutes made from soy or tofu.

- Soy additives found in more than 60% of processed foods including textured soy protein (50–70% soy protein) added to hotdogs, hamburgers, sausages and other meat products; soy protein isolate (90% soy protein) used in energy bars, sports drinks, cereals, granola bars, imitation dairy products, ice cream, cheese and even doughnuts [78].

Add Lignans

Plant lignans are a type of dietary fiber that gut bacteria convert into weak estrogen-like compounds (phytoestrogens). Foods containing lignans appear to decrease estrogen levels, delay the onset of diabetes, and reduce diet-induced fat accumulation [79].

Lignans are found in many fiber-rich foods such as berries, seeds (particularly flaxseeds and sesame seeds), grains, nuts and fruits. Consider having some lignans every day, if you are not eating them routinely.

Influencing Estrogen Metabolism

Gut bacteria convert estrogen into a number of different metabolites. Estrogen metabolites have different health effects and remain in the body for different time periods.

Two common estrogen metabolites with very different health effects are:

- Active metabolite (16alpha-OHE1) that is longer acting and associated with weight gain, or

- Inactive metabolite (2-OHE1) associated with reduced body fat and increased lean body mass [80].

Diet, lifestyle, weight, and genetic factors (including factors related to race/ethnicity) influence the mix of gut bacteria, which estrogen metabolites are more commonly produced, and blood estrogen levels (as discussed above). Eating more berries, fruits, vegetables, herbs and spices, containing polyphenols, as well as decreasing smoking, caffeine intake, and body size may help increase the proportion of the more beneficial metabolite [81].

Eating to Starve Lipedema Fat and Excess Estrogen

To summarize:

- Estrogen and related hormones are major factors in lipedema fat accumulation and many other conditions.

- Gut dysbiosis interferes with estrogen regulation; correcting dysbiosis should help normalize blood estrogen levels.

- Foods from animal sources contain estrogens and cholesterol, which can be converted into estrogen.

- Food choices may increase the proportion of beneficial estrogen metabolites.

- Salt intake should be monitored to stay within the recommended range (see "Sodium" on page 79).

Eat foods that support normal estrogen levels and overall health:

- Colorful vegetables, fruits, herbs, and spices containing anti-angiogenic and anti-oxidant factors.

- Lignans in flaxseeds, sesame seeds, other seeds, berries, or nuts.

- Omega-3 fats and other anti-inflammatory foods.

- Organic soybeans and tofu.

- Fermented foods including fermented soy.

Starve lipedema fat, excess estrogen, and gut dysbiosis:

- Limit foods from animal sources.

- Avoid meats with added estrogen, such as conventional (not organic) beef. Eat grass-fed meats in moderation.

- Avoid foods made with processed soy or soy additives.

Endocrine Disruptors

Estrogen-like endocrine disrupting chemicals (EEDC) are synthetic chemicals found in foods and food containers that interfere with estrogen activity. For example, pesticides, BPA and other brominated diphenyl esters, PCBs (polychlorinated biphenyls), and phthalates.

EEDC affect the synthesis, metabolism, binding, transport and cellular responses to natural estrogens primarily by interfering with binding to cellular receptors that are normally activated by estrogen. Females exposed to EEDC may develop early (precocious puberty), have reproductive disorders of the ovary (aneuploidy, polycystic ovary syndrome, and altered menstrual cycles) and uterus (endometriosis, uterine fibroids), or cancer of the breast or reproductive system [82].

Minimize EEDC exposure by selecting organic foods not treated with pesticides, minimizing the use of plastics for food storage, and selecting canned goods in BPA-free cans.

Chapter 3

Recommended Eating Pattern

Eat primarily whole foods, mostly plants, including a wide variety of rainbow-colored vegetables and fruits, as well as fermented foods. Use herbs and spices to provide your favorite flavors.

Starve lymphedema and lipedema by avoiding added sugars (especially fructose), refined grains (especially grains containing gluten), and chemically modified fats. Limit animal products and high-salt foods. Avoiding dairy (other than kefir and yogurt) appears to help with lipedema.

Whole foods are best because most prepared foods contain added sugar, salt, soy, unhealthy fats, or undesirable additives. Juicing (other than green vegetable juices) is only recommended for those who cannot eat solid food because juicing breaks down fiber, removing an important nutritional and digestive health benefit. Fruit juices should be minimized because they raise blood glucose more rapidly than whole fruit.

Modify this eating pattern if you are vegetarian, vegan, gluten intolerant, have food allergies, diabetes, or other dietary concerns.

Foods are grouped by recommended frequency:

- Eat Primarily: have a variety of different foods from this list every day in reasonable serving sizes. Include at least a half-cup of beans, a half-cup of whole grains (such as oats) or starchy vegetables, and one cup of fruit (preferably citrus and banana) each day.

- Eat in Limited Quantities: foods best enjoyed in smaller amounts and only a few times a week, including no more than 6-8 servings of animal products each week. Servings are 3-4 ounces of cooked meat, 2 eggs, 8 ounces of milk, or 1.5 ounces of cheese.

- Eat Rarely or Never: save these for special occasions, if you still want them.

The lists below can help you make better food choices. For those who want more detail, we explain major nutrients in Chapter 4, other nutritional factors in Chapter 5, and provide a shopping guide in Appendix A.

If this very different from what you eat now, start with 'Eat Primarily' foods for 6-8 weeks; then add foods from the two other categories and see how they work for you. See Chapter 7 for help changing your eating pattern.

Eat Primarily

- Vegetables with bright colors and flavors such as dark green leafy vegetables, colorful beets, corn, squash, peppers, and flavorful onions, garlic, mushrooms, and herbs.

- Beans, legumes or pulses: such as adzuki beans, black beans, butter beans (gigantes), cannellini beans, chickpeas (garbanzo or ceci beans), fava beans, great northern beans, kidney beans, lentils, lima beans, peas, navy beans, pinto beans, etc.

- Berries (fresh or frozen): blackberries, blueberries, cranberries, raspberries, strawberries, etc.

- Citrus fruits: grapefruit, orange, etc.

- Fruits: apples, apricots, bananas, cherries, grapes, kiwi fruit, mangoes, melons, papaya, peaches, pears, pineapple, plums, etc.

- Potatoes: smaller waxy potatoes such as new, red, purple, etc. Not starchy Russet or Idaho potatoes.

- Sweet potatoes or yams.

- Grains (whole grains not containing gluten): amaranth, brown rice, buckwheat, millet, oats, quinoa, sorghum, teff, and wild rice.

- Fermented foods: kefir and yogurt with active cultures, sauerkraut, dill or sour pickles (subject to salt limits), kimchi, etc.

- Soy that is minimally processed or fermented: soybeans/edamame), tofu, miso, natto, tempeh.

- Milks (unsweetened non-dairy milk drinks): almond milk, coconut milk, or hemp milk.

- Coffee, tea (black, green, herbal, red, white), unsweetened cocoa or cacao.

- Other: ground flaxseed, avocados, olives, coconut, coconut milk, spices.

Eat in Limited Quantities

- Brazil nuts: Brazil nuts are high in selenium which can help reduce swelling but excess selenium can cause health issues [83]. Either eat limited quantities of Brazil nuts (1 ounce or 6 nuts purchased shelled, or 3 nuts purchased unshelled per day) OR take a selenium supplement, not both.

- Chocolate: dark chocolate with 70% or more cacao.

- Dairy (preferably organic, not recommended for lipedema): butter or ghee (clarified butter), cheeses (not processed cheeses or cheese spreads), goat's milk cheese (goat cheese), sheep's milk cheese, milk.

- Eggs including yolks: preferably organic, pastured or free-range

- Fish: tuna, wild salmon, mackerel, herring, sardines, anchovies, and other seafood high in omega-3 unsaturated fats.

- Meats: preferably organic grass-fed beef, buffalo, lamb, pork, wild game.

- Poultry: preferably organic chicken (without skin), turkey, duck including dark meat.

- Nuts and seeds (raw and unsalted): almonds, cashews, hazelnuts, macadamia nuts, pecans, pistachios, pumpkin seeds, sesame seeds, sunflower seeds, walnuts.

- Oils: extra-virgin olive, avocado, walnut, coconut, cocoa butter, flaxseed, macadamia, sesame oil.

- Salad dressing products containing healthy fats and modest amounts of sodium or sweeteners.

- Sugar and real maple syrup.

- Condiments: chili, hot sauce, or pepper sauce, horseradish, mustard, salsa, tamari soy sauce, tapenade, vinegar (white, red wine, apple cider, balsamic), Worcestershire sauce, etc.

- Dried fruits: cranberries (low sugar), currants, dates, figs, prunes, raisins.

- Wine: preferably red, no more than 3 servings (5 ounces or 150 ml)/ week.

Eat Rarely or Never

- Grain products containing gluten (wheat, barley or rye): breads, breakfast cereals, bulgur, cakes, cookies, couscous, crackers, cupcakes, kamut, noodles, pancakes, pasta, pies, pita, pizza, triticale, waffles, etc.

- Gluten-free food substitutes: breads, pasta, pizza, baked goods, etc. made with cornstarch, potato starch, rice starch, tapioca starch, etc.

- Fried foods and food products such as chips, crisps, fries, etc.

- Meat processed or preserved using nitrates, nitrites, or salt (such as hot dogs or lunch meats), cooked at high temperatures, or over a flame.

- Meat substitutes made from gluten, seitan, or highly processed soy.

- Soy-based processed foods: infant formula, soymilk, etc.

- Sugary snacks: candies, energy bars, fruit roll-ups, ice cream, sherbet, etc.

- Sugary sweeteners: agave syrup or nectar, high-fructose corn syrup, honey, and artificial sweeteners.

- Sweet condiments: chutney, jams, jellies, preserves, sauces, syrups, etc.

- Sweet drinks, sugar sweetened and diet (artificially sweetened): sodas, soft drinks, teas and tea-based beverages, coffee and coffee-based beverages, energy drinks, fruit drinks (especially 100% fruit drinks), etc.

- Unhealthy fats: hydrogenated oils (palm, palm kernel), polyunsaturated oils (corn, cottonseed, grape seed, safflower, soybean, sunflower), trans-fats, and chemically modified fats. Includes regular and vegan mayonnaise.

- Beer, liquor, mixed drinks, wine coolers, etc.

Chapter **4:**

Food Label Nutrients

Food label information can help you make better choices. In this chapter, we explain major nutrients (macronutrients), the useful parts of food labels, and what to look for when comparing foods. The next chapter covers other nutritional factors not shown on food labels.

Fat, carbohydrate, and protein–as defined and explained below–summarize the nutritional value of foods and the amount of energy provided (calories). While these values are important, labels do not tell the whole story about food desirability.

Use food labels together with our recommended food lists and shopping guide:

- Whole foods and fresh foods (not packaged) may not have nutrition labels.

- Recommended foods–including anti-angiogenic foods–may contain little fat, carbohydrate, or protein. These foods provide important nutritional benefits other than calories and should be a major part of your eating plan.

- Carbohydrate type is more important than quantity. We recommend natural sugars or starches (complex carbohydrates) and avoid refined carbohydrates.

- Fat types are also important: some fats are beneficial while others harmful, as explained below.

In terms of major nutrients, our whole foods and plant based eating pattern is:

- High in carbohydrates, specifically complex carbohydrates from vegetables, beans, and whole grains plus natural sugars from fruit.

- Low fat, with most fats from plants and limited fat from animal products.

- Lower in protein with most protein from plant sources.

Changing to our recommended eating pattern means replacing processed foods with whole foods including vegetables, beans, whole grains, and fruits, and healthy fats. Animal products are optional and limited in terms of serving sizes and frequency.

Conventional Western diets and our whole food plant based eating plan are both high-carb with the majority of calories from carbohydrates. However, the types of carbohydrates included, and their metabolic effects, are very different.

Most carbohydrates in Western diets are highly refined sweets and grain products. Sweets include sweetened drinks, fruit juices, candies, desserts, etc. Many sweets contain concentrated fructose.

Grain products include breads, pasta, pizza, cereal, baked goods, snack foods, beer, etc. as well as processed or prepared foods made with flour. Most Americans get more than half of their calories from wheat flour. Many grain-based food products are also high in sugar, salt, and unhealthy fats (chemically modified fats).

Our recommended eating plan replaces refined carbohydrates with whole foods containing starches, or complex carbohydrates, and natural sugars. Starches include beans, starchy vegetables (potatoes, corn, etc.), and whole grains. Natural sugars are found in vegetables, fruits, and dairy products.

These types of carbohydrates have very different metabolic effects:

- Refined carbohydrates raise blood glucose levels very quickly, triggering a chain of metabolic effects (described above) that contribute to inflammation, obesity, fatty liver disease and diabetes.

- Starches are digested more slowly, resulting in a smaller increase in blood glucose over a longer time. This avoids the rebound hunger and low blood sugar (hypoglycemia) that can result following a refined carbohydrate meal.

- Natural sugars produce a moderate increase in blood glucose.

A variety of eating patterns can improve lymphedema and lipedema including:

- Vegetarian or vegan: plant products only.

- Ovo-lacto vegetarian: plants, eggs, dairy but not meat.

- Pescetarian: fish, possibly other seafood, and plants; may include eggs or dairy.

- Low carbohydrate, or very low-carbohydrate ketogenic diet (also known as Atkins or Banting diet): most calories come from fats; carbohydrates provide less than 25% of calories.

- Paleo: meat, fish, eggs, vegetables, and fruit; no dairy, grains, or processed foods.

Common features of beneficial eating patterns include:

- Whole foods with minimal processing in place of processed foods, prepared foods, or fast food.

- Eliminating sugars from simple carbohydrates including concentrated fructose, and refined grain-based foods including gluten.

- Carbohydrates from starches (complex carbohydrates) including vegetables, beans, whole grains and fruit.

- Balancing calories with metabolic needs and activity level to avoid over nutrition.

- Fats that are health supporting, avoiding unhealthy fats (explained below).

- Sodium: keeping salt or sodium intake within a healthy range.

These eating patterns differ in how they disrupt the fat and sugar combination responsible for gut dysbiosis, endotoxins, systemic inflammation, and other negative health effects (described in Chapter 2):

- Whole food plant based, vegetarian, vegan, ovo-lacto vegetarian, and pescetarian diets reduce sugars (complex carbohydrates only) and tightly limit fats. Animal fats are either excluded (vegan) or restricted in terms of quantity and frequency of fat-containing meals.

- Low carbohydrate and paleo diets tightly limit sugars (carbohydrates are the source of sugars) but are high in fats. Fats become an energy source based on ketones in place of glucose.

In terms of overall health and other health conditions, a whole food, plant-based approach has stronger and more extensive research support, especially with regard to heart disease, fatty liver disease, and metabolic syndrome/diabetes. For a good summary of the research on 15 different conditions,

---

Ketogenic Diets

Human metabolism changes while fasting or if carbohydrate intake falls below about 25% of required calories or 130 grams per day (your mileage may vary). After glycogen stores are exhausted, the body starts converting stored fat to glucose as a source of energy and the liver releases ketones, an alternative energy source for the brain (which is unable to convert fats) and muscles.

Low carbohydrate diets are called ketogenic diets because they promote a low level of ketone release and fat mobilization by limiting carbohydrates. A ketogenic diet is very different from diabetic ketoacidosis, a life-threatening condition where the lack of insulin triggers the release of toxic quantities of ketones and ketoacids in someone with insulin dependent diabetes.

A low carbohydrate or very low-carbohydrate ketogenic eating pattern promotes short term weight reduction, which provides some benefit for people with lymphedema or lipedema. However, a meta-analysis of large cohort studies concluded that low-carbohydrate diets are likely unsafe because they significantly increased risk of all-cause mortality compared to conventional Western diets [84].

see **How Not to Die** by Michael Greger, MD, and Gene Stone (Flatiron Books 2015).

Reading Food Labels

American food labels have a box labeled Nutrition Facts similar to the examples in Figure 4-1 on page 70. These are the most important items and we explain them below:

- Serving Size and Servings per Container

- Calories

- Total Fat

- Cholesterol

- Sodium

- Total Carbohydrate or Total Carbs

- Protein

Look for nutrient amounts in grams (g) or milligrams (mg); the percentage values are not useful.

Serving Size

Labels show nutrient information for one serving, the serving size, and the number of servings per container. Nutrient values are shown as the amount per serving. Look closely at the serving size definition because one serving can be surprisingly small, compared to what you might eat in one sitting. For example, a small bag of chips may contain 3 servings, or a packaged entrée may provide 4 servings, according to the label.

Multi-serving packages may show nutritional information for a whole package as well as per serving. Labels for foods frequently eaten in combinations (such as cereal and milk) or mixes where you add ingredients (such as cake mix where you add eggs, water, and oil) may provide details for the combination and for package contents alone.

To evaluate the nutrient content of your portion (the quantity you plan to eat), determine the equivalent number of servings (as given on the label), and multiply the number of servings times the nutrient quantity per serving.

For example, if you are planning to eat a package of soup that contains two servings, and each serving is 15g of carbohydrate, your portion is 15*2 or 30g of carbohydrate.

Tip: Google or other search engines will convert units and calculate quantities. For example, searching for '100 grams to oz' will return 3.5 ounces. You can also search for nutritional information, for example 'grapefruit carbs.' Searching is convenient, but the results may not be accurate due to product variations.

Figure 4-1: Nutrition Facts Label

Nutrition Facts

Serving Size 2/3 cup (55g)
Servings Per Container About 8

Amount Per Serving

Calories 230	Calories from Fat 72

	% Daily Value*
Total Fat 8g	**12%**
Saturated Fat 1g	**5%**
Trans Fat 0g	
Cholesterol 0mg	**0%**
Sodium 160mg	**7%**
Total Carbohydrate 37g	**12%**
Dietary Fiber 4g	**16%**
Sugars 1g	
Protein 3g	

Vitamin A	10%
Vitamin C	8%
Calcium	20%
Iron	45%

* Percent Daily Values are based on a 2,000 calorie diet. Your daily value may be higher or lower depending on your calorie needs.

	Calories:	2,000	2,500
Total Fat	Less than	65g	80g
Sat Fat	Less than	20g	25g
Cholesterol	Less than	300mg	300mg
Sodium	Less than	2,400mg	2,400mg
Total Carbohydrate		300g	375g
Dietary Fiber		25g	30g

Nutrition Facts

8 servings per container

Serving size   2/3 cup (55g)

Amount per 2/3 cup

Calories   230

% DV*

12%	**Total Fat** 8g
5%	Saturated Fat 1g
	Trans Fat 0g
0%	**Cholesterol** 0mg
7%	**Sodium** 160mg
12%	**Total Carbs** 37g
14%	Dietary Fiber 4g
	Sugars 1g
	Added Sugars 0g
	Protein 3g

10%	**Vitamin D** 2mcg
20%	**Calcium** 260mg
45%	**Iron** 8mg
5%	**Potassium** 235mg

* Footnote on Daily Values (DV) and calories reference to be inserted here.

Ingredient List

In addition to reading the nutritional information, check the ingredient list so you know what you are really eating. Ingredients are shown in order by quantity, starting with ingredients used in the largest amount (by weight) and ending with the smallest amounts.

What to look for

If you have food allergies or sensitivities, it is not safe to rely on the list of allergens on the label, also check the ingredient. American labeling requirements only include proteins from eight common food allergens.

A list of ingredients to minimize or avoid is in Appendix B. This list includes:

- Additives: chemicals added to processed foods to improve flavor, texture, or stability that can increase inflammation or disrupt metabolic signaling in some individuals [85]. For example, monosodium glutamate (MSG).

- Artificial Sweeteners, see "Artificial Sweeteners" on page 90.

- Grains/Gluten, see "Grain and Gluten Metabolism" on page 35.

- Soy: processed soy products, see "Moderate Plant-Based Estrogens from Soy" on page 54.

- Sugars: all types of natural sweeteners, see "Sugars" on page 82.

- Undesirable fats, see "Trans-Fats and Chemically Modified Fats" on page 77.

Calories

Calories measure the energy provided by one serving of food as fuel for your body. Calories are not nutrients, per se, but a measure of the energy provided by the major nutrients. Calories are calculated from the amount of fat, carbohydrate and protein in a serving using the conversion factors in Table 4-1: Macronutrient Energy Density.

Tracking energy input in calories and energy usage in calories provides a way to compare what you eat against what your body actually uses.

Healthy eating includes balancing energy input (food calories consumed) with energy usage (food calories burned) on a daily basis. Our bodies thriftily convert excess calories (from any nutrient, especially carbohydrates and fat) into fat for storage. Excess calories (over nutrition) cause unhealthy changes in gut bacteria and contributes to diabetes and other health issues.

Daily energy usage includes:

- Resting metabolic rate (RMR): the energy our bodies use at rest, while not doing other activities. RMR can be measured using a special instrument or estimated based on height and weight.

- Non-exercise activity thermogenesis (NEAT): energy our bodies use during activities of daily living including working, playing, and dancing (but not exercise) can vary by up to 2,000 calories per day. Inactivity contributes to weight gain and spending more time standing or walking helps reverse this trend; research show that obese individuals spend 2.5 more hours per day sitting than their sedentary but lean counterparts [86].

- Exercise: energy used for activities to develop or maintain fitness such as power-walking, jogging, running, biking, team sports, etc.

Table 4-1: Macronutrient Energy Density

Macronutrient	Calories/gram
Fat	9
Carbohydrate	4
Protein	4

Consult a registered dietitian for help evaluating your energy usage, setting goals for energy intake, and developing a personalized eating plan.

Tracking calorie intake compared to daily energy usage can help you decide if you need to change your eating pattern and what changes to make. Special apps or online tools make the tracking process easier. Some tools can look-up nutritional information by scanning food product bar codes. See "Food Diary" on page 226 for more information. Tracking net carbohydrates may be easier than calorie counting for tracking and meal planning (see "Carbo-hydrate Counting" on page 226).

What to look for

- We look more at carbohydrates and sugars than calories, as explained below.

- If two alternatives are otherwise acceptable, the lower calorie food is probably better for you.

Total Fat

Foods containing fat include anything made with meat, eggs, animal fats (lard, tallow, etc.), dairy products, oils, nuts, and seeds. Certain types of fat are necessary for health (the essential fatty acids) and others are good sources of nutrition, but some types of fat can be harmful.

Fats provide more than twice as much food energy (calories) per gram as protein or carbohydrates. Fatty foods can be tasty and filling. Fat provides a long-lasting feeling of satiety without causing rapid increases in blood glucose.

Chemically, fats are compounds (triglycerides) with three fatty acid chains connected to a glycerol backbone. Our bodies build up energy reserves by accumulating triglycerides in many locations, including fat depots (adipose tissue).

Fats are classified based on two properties:

- Molecule size or the number of carbon atoms in the fatty acid chain: short-, medium-, or long-chain fats. Foods contain mixtures of chain lengths and the majority of food fats are long-chain fats but certain foods contain primarily short- or medium-chain fats.

- Stability of the chemical structure: saturated fats are solid at room temperature and chemically very stable because they have hydrogen atoms in all possible binding positions. Unsaturated fats (also known as monounsaturated or polyunsaturated fats) are liquids at room temperature and less stable because they have unused binding positions where hydrogen or oxygen can attach.

Saturated fats include solid fats in meats and dairy products, coconut oil, and cocoa butter. Hydrogenated vegetable oils and similar chemically modified fats are saturated by adding hydrogen to unsaturated oils.

Oils or fats from plants (nuts and seeds), egg yolks, and fatty fish are mostly unsaturated fats. Other seafood and animal products contain mixtures of saturated and unsaturated fats in different proportions.

Essential fats are specific unsaturated fats humans cannot synthesize internally and must obtain from food sources to remain healthy. We explain these fats in the next chapter because they do not appear on nutrition labels (see "Omega-3 vs. Omega-6 Fats" on page 85).

Table 4-2 shows example fats and fatty foods in each part of our recommended eating pattern.

Each type of fat affects the body differently as explained below:

- Saturated fats from animal sources can be healthy in moderation.
- Trans-fats and chemically modified fats should be avoided for good health.
- Short and medium-chain fats can be especially beneficial.

Saturated Fats

Saturated fats have been linked to heart disease leading to recommendations for a low fat, high-carbohydrate diet. Newer research shows that replacing fats with refined carbohydrates increases health risks and obesity, and saturated fats can be part of a healthy eating pattern. For example, a large study showed that risk of heart disease was lower for those who ate more saturated fat; specifically dairy fat was associated with lower heart disease risk, meat fat was associated with slightly increased risk, while butter and plant fats did not affect risk [87].

Table 4-2: Recommended Fats and Fatty Foods

Fat Type (Primary)	Eat Primarily	Eat in Limited Quantities	Eat Rarely or Never
Unsaturated Fats	Avocados	Eggs, Nuts, Olive Oil	
• Omega-3	Chia Seeds, Flaxseed, Walnuts	Fish	
• Omega-6	Soy	Sunflower Seeds	Corn Oil, Cottonseed Oil, Grape Seed Oil, Safflower Oil, Soybean Oil, Sunflower Oil
Saturated Fats			
• Short-, Medium-Chain	Coconut Oil	Butter, Ghee, Goat Cheese, Sheep's Milk Cheese	Palm Oil, Palm Kernel Oil
• Long-Chain	Kefir, Yogurt	Cheese, Chocolate, Milk, Poultry, Red Meats	
Trans-Fats			Hydrogenated Oils, Margarine, Shortening
Chemically Modified Fats			Interesterified Oils

Our recommended eating pattern replaces refined carbohydrates with complex carbohydrates and natural sugars. Overall fat level is low and we emphasize healthier fats, especially omega-3 fats and medium-chain fats. For some people this will mean eating more fat from fish, eggs, beans, nuts, seeds, avocados, and coconut.

People with lymphedema may want to avoid certain animal products:

- Fats in dairy products and red meats should be avoided or only eaten occasionally in modest quantities because they contribute to the growth of E. coli and other gram-negative obesogenic gut microbes.

- Infants and children with lymphatic malformations may have trouble metabolizing long-chain fats and require a special diet based on medium-chain fats from MCT oil.

- Lymphatic overload and chyle leakage (chylous ascites or chylothorax) may be improved by avoiding high-fat foods containing mostly long-chain fats, to reduce the volume of chyle.

- High salt animal products including processed or preserved meats, certain types of cheeses, poultry injected with salt solution or broth during processing, roasted chickens and other prepared meats injected with salt water, and brined, marinated, or sauced meat dishes.

- Grain-fed meat and dairy products are less desirable than grass-fed meats and organic dairy products because the grain-fed foods contain primarily omega-6 fats. See "Omega-3 vs. Omega-6 Fats" on page 85.

- Farmed fish have more omega-6 fats and less omega-3 fats than wild fish, because they are grain-fed.

Diets high in saturated fats increase the risk of skin infections by reducing sebum content, drying the skin, and inhibiting the acid barrier (increasing skin pH) [88]. This is an area for further research and may relate to mix of omega-3 and omega-6 fats in these diets.

Trans-Fats and Chemically Modified Fats

Fast food, fried foods, snack foods, candy, processed foods, industrially produced frozen, canned and baked goods, baking mixes, frosting, etc. should be avoided for several reasons—including the types of fat they contain. Until recently, many of these products contained hydrogenated oils containing harmful trans-fats [89].

Since the FDA banned trans-fats, hydrogenated oils are being replaced by combinations of palm oil, chemically modified fats (primarily interesterified soybean oil), and emulsifiers with little research into the health implications of these new ingredients. Interesterified fats are chemically modified to change the melting point and slow spoilage. Food labels do not identify fats modified by interesterification. Interesterified fats can have negative health effects in high doses [90].

Hydrogenated vegetable oils in commercial food fryers are being replaced by regular soybean oil that may not be healthier. Regular oil oxidizes more easily than hydrogenated oil. After being heated for several hours, soybean oil forms toxic compounds (such as 4-Hydroxy-2-trans-nonenal or HNE) absorbed by fried foods [91].

What to look for

- Trans-fats: 0 grams per serving.

- No unhealthy fat ingredients; check the list of ingredients to avoid in Appendix B.

Short and Medium-Chain Fats

Many foods contain fats with different chain lengths but most foods are primarily long-chain fats. The exceptions include:

- Coconut oil and MCT oil (medium chain-triglyceride oil) derived from coconuts that are primarily medium-chain fats.

- Goats' milk and cheeses made with milk from goats or sheep are high in medium-chain fats.

- Butter and ghee are primarily short-chain fats.

Chain length affects the way the body metabolizes fats:

- Long-chain fats are absorbed via lymphatic villi from cells lining the small intestine and pass through the lymphatic system before entering the bloodstream.

- Medium- and short-chain fats enter the blood stream in the intestines and go directly into the liver via the portal vein. Medium- and short-chain fats are converted to energy more quickly and efficiently than long-chain fats.

Coconut oil can be used in cooking or baking as a healthy alternative to shortening containing chemically modified fats, although some people dislike the taste or smell. Replace shortening or butter with an equal quantity of coconut oil.

Cholesterol

Cholesterol is a waxy, fat-like substance found in all cells of the body (in small quantities) and in plaque that can build up inside arteries causing atherosclerosis and coronary artery disease. Cholesterol is used to synthesize hormones (including estrogen in premenopausal women), vitamin D, and substances that help you digest foods. Typically one-third of the cholesterol in the body comes from foods containing animal fats and the other two-thirds is synthesized within the body [92].

Over half of the cholesterol in the American diet come from eggs and egg mixed dishes, chicken and chicken mixed dishes, beef and beef mixed dishes, burgers, and regular cheese [93].

What to look for

- Look for the alternative with the least cholesterol.

Sodium

Salt or sodium chloride provides sodium, an essential mineral, and possibly iodine and other minerals. Excessive sodium intake contributes to lymphedema, high blood pressure (hypertension) in susceptible people, and other disorders. Many people get high amounts of sodium from salty, processed, prepared and preserved foods, without adding salt at the table.

Keeping salt intake consistently low (between 500 and 1,500 mg/day) and increasing potassium intake from vegetables and fruits will help improve both blood and lymph circulation [94]. This means limiting fast food, processed foods, salty foods, meats injected or cured with salt, sauces, packaged salad dressings, etc. Taste your food before adding salt at the table, and add the minimum amount.

Note: carbohydrate reduction affects sodium metabolism and additional salt in the form of broth or soup may be recommended if you are on a low carbohydrate or ketogenic diet. Consult a registered dietitian who is experienced with these eating plans for a personalized recommendation, especially if you have salt-sensitive hypertension or are take diuretics.

What to look for

- Pink salt, Himalayan salt, or sea salt contain more trace minerals, are not as highly refined, and may taste better than conventional table salt. Kosher salt has larger crystals; it is not a different kind of salt.

- When comparing sodium levels in products, look for the alternative with the lowest sodium.

Total Carbohydrate/Total Carbs

Carbohydrate information on food labels includes:

- Total Carbohydrate or Total Carbs: total weight for all types of carbohydrate (explained below) and dietary fiber per serving.

- Dietary Fiber: amount of fiber per serving (if any). As explained below, fiber provides important health benefits, even if we cannot digest it.

- Sugars: grams of simple sugars per serving, including the added sugars.

- Added Sugars (optional, not on all labels): grams of sugars added during processing.

Carbohydrates are converted into glucose (blood sugar) by digestion and provide the primary source of energy for the body. Excess glucose can be stored in the liver as glycogen, a fast-acting energy reserve. When both glucose and insulin levels are high, the liver will convert glucose to fat (see "Fatty Liver Disease" on page 41).

There are three types of carbohydrates:

- Refined carbohydrates are the most common carbohydrates in the Western diet and include all types of processed sugars or sweeteners, and refined starches such as flour milled from wheat or other grains.

- Natural sugars: found in fruits, vegetables, and dairy products. Includes fruit sugar (fructose), milk sugar (lactose), other types of sugars.

- Starches or complex carbohydrates combine complex sugar molecules and fiber: starchy vegetables like potatoes and corn, beans (legumes), brown rice and other whole grains.

The label item for Sugars includes sugar molecules from refined carbohydrates, natural sugars, and added sugars. These are termed simple carbohydrates or simple sugars because they contain small sugar molecules that can be digested quickly.

Starches have a complex structure including very long chains of sugar molecules folded together and encased in protein or fiber. Before sugar molecules can be absorbed, the outer casing must be removed, the chain unfolded, and the individual molecules broken apart. This process takes time, which slows the absorption of sugars and provides a sustained release of energy and a longer-term, moderate increase in blood sugar after a meal.

When starchy food ingredients are processed, these large molecules are broken apart, sugar molecules are recombined into smaller chains, and the fiber may be removed. The resulting food product contains starches that are digested more easily and increase blood sugar quickly, like a simple carbohydrate.

Total Carbohydrate values can be misleading because they include non-nutritive fiber. Net carbohydrates, or available carbohydrates are a more useful value calculated by subtracting fiber grams from total carbohydrate grams (see "Carbohydrate Counting" on page 226). For example, one serving of oat crackers contains 21 grams of total carbohydrate, 4 grams of fiber, and 6 grams of protein, Subtracting 4 from 21 gives 17 grams of net carbohydrate per serving.

Subtracting the sugars from the net carbohydrates gives the starch or complex carbohydrate content. Continuing the oat cracker example, 17 grams of net carbohydrate less 4 grams of sugars per serving gives 13 grams of starch or complex carbohydrate per serving.

You may not need to plan or track calories or carbohydrates if you choose foods based on our recommended eating plan. However, you may need to plan carbs if you have diabetes or you may want to track carbs while making changes in your eating pattern.

Use these guidelines if you need to plan your carbohydrate intake:

- If you eat meat and dairy products (within our recommended limits), plan on 65% of total calories from carbohydrates.

- Without animal products, plan on 80% of total calories from carbohydrates.

- Multiply your desired daily calories by the percentage given above. For example, 2,000 calories per day without animal products would be 80% or 1,600 calories per day from carbohydrates (the remaining calories are fat and protein).

- Convert calories to grams of carbohydrate by dividing by 4 calories per gram. Continuing the same example: 1,600 calories is 400 grams of carbohydrate per day.

Consult your health care provider and a registered dietitian (see www.eatright.org) for help designing a meal plan that is appropriate for you.

Anyone taking insulin or other diabetes medication should coordinate with their health care provider to adjust these medications when changing carbohydrate intake. This includes changing the type of carbohydrate as well as quantities because each type of carbohydrate affects blood glucose levels and insulin requirements differently.

Dietary Fiber

Fiber is only found in plant-based foods and includes molecules in vegetables, fruits, whole grains, and beans that we are not able to digest completely. Labels on foods with less than one gram of fiber per serving may say "Not a significant source of dietary fiber."

Dietary fiber provides many health benefits and supports health promoting gut microbiota by increasing helpful bacteria (see "Inulin" on page 87) and bacterial diversity. Fiber also helps regulate appetite and digestion.

Processed foods contain less fiber than whole foods because processing breaks down fiber and reduces its beneficial effects. For example, making flour from wheat, high fructose syrup from corn, soy isolate from soybeans, sugar from sugar cane or sugar beets, juice from fruits or vegetables, etc. High-fiber processed foods are often fortified with food additives providing little nutritional benefit such as cellulose (from cotton or wood), oat hull fiber, wheat fiber, etc.

What to look for

Desirability of fiber depends upon the product:

- Whole foods: naturally occurring fiber is good and more may be better.

- Processed or prepared foods: natural fiber is good; added fiber from food additives are less desirable and can affect taste. Compare the ingredients on the label to the list of food additives in Appendix B.

Sugars

Sugars are the simple carbohydrate portion of the Total Carbohydrates including naturally occurring sugars and added sugars (which may or may not be shown on the label).

All nutritive sweeteners are combinations of three simple sugar molecules: glucose (or dextrose), fructose and galactose. Glucose is immediately usable as a source of energy but fructose and galactose must be converted into glucose by the liver before they can be used.

Common forms of sugar are pairs of these molecules. For example, table sugar (sucrose) combines fructose and glucose, and milk sugar (lactose) found in dairy products is galactose and glucose.

Fructose (and other sugars) can also be converted into fat by the liver, which contributes to fatty liver disease (see "Fatty Liver Disease" on page 41). Fructose can cause weight gain and elevated fat levels (blood triglycerides) as part of an eating pattern that provides more calories than required (over nutrition) [95].

Added Sugars

Some labels show a value for Added Sugars separately. This includes all types of sweetener added during processing, not just sugar. There are many names for sugar and other sweeteners; these are included in the list of ingredients to avoid in Appendix B.

Having added sugars on the label makes it easier to identify unexpected sources of sugar. For example, some varieties of canned beans have sugar added.

What to look for

• Look for the option with lowest net carbohydrates (Total Carbohydrates minus Fiber).

• If Added Sugars are given, look for the option with the smallest amount. Whole foods will not have added sugars.

Protein

Our bodies use protein as building blocks for muscle and other types of tissues or as a source of energy. Proteins come from plants including beans, legumes, soy, nuts, vegetables, and whole grains as well as from animal products like meats, eggs, and dairy foods. Fruits contain very little protein and foods that are primarily sugars (simple carbohydrates) or fats do not provide any protein.

Humans and plant-eating animals make proteins from the amino acids contained in plants. Vegetables provide all the proteins and amino acids humans require; we do not have a biological need for meat or eggs.

Plant proteins are 'incomplete proteins' because no single plant provides all nine indispensable amino acids. However, each family of plants has different amino acids and eating a variety of plant foods every day provides all nine amino acids.

Many people are concerned about getting 'enough' protein or think more protein might provide health benefits. Protein deficiency is extremely rare–anyone getting enough nutrition to avoid wasting away is getting adequate protein.

Protein requirements are based on muscle mass (lean body mass) and are higher during periods of rapid growth. Body fat accumulation does not increase the need for dietary protein without muscle growth.

Recommended daily intake for protein is 46 grams/day for women (71 grams/day during pregnancy and lactation) or 56 grams/day for men [96]. In America, women average 150% of the recommended amount (68.1 grams/day) and men average 175% (98.8 grams/day) [97]. Excess protein does not improve health. On the contrary, excess protein makes certain conditions worse, such as chronic kidney disease, and excess calories (from all types of nutrients) contribute to obesity.

Sometimes people with lymphedema think if they stop eating protein they will have less protein in their tissue fluid and reduce their risk of lymphedema infections. Eating less protein does not affect protein in the tissue fluid. Not eating adequate protein, or more commonly, not being able to digest proteins, can result in swelling (edema) from protein deficiency malnutrition.

Protein is about 10-15% of calories in a whole-food plant based eating pattern. Protein intake is not a concern for anyone who is eating a variety of vegetables including beans, whole grains, and nuts.

What to look for

- When comparing foods where other values are comparable, more protein may be better.

Chapter 5

Other Nutritional Factors

This chapter covers other important nutritional factors including:

- Omega-3 fats that fight inflammation and omega-6 fats that promote inflammation.

- Inulin, a specific type of fiber with important benefits.

- Fermented foods support healthy gut microbes and stimulate the immune system.

- Artificial sweeteners you may want to avoid.

Omega-3 vs. Omega-6 Fats

Omega-3 and omega-6 fats are both required but have different health effects. Most people will benefit from increasing omega-3 fats or supplements and reducing omega-6 fat intake.

Both omega-3 and omega-6 fats are essential fatty acids because humans cannot synthesize them from other sources and must get these fats from food. Fats are required for cell membranes, skin integrity, cellular communication, immune system regulation, and the development of nerves, eyes and the brain [98].

Omega-3 fats are especially important for anyone with lymphedema because these fats become part of the acid barrier that protects the skin from infections [99].

Omega-3 fats are anti-angiogenic factors and anti-inflammatory while omega-6 fats are pro-inflammatory. Fighting inflammation requires changing the ratio of omega-6 to omega-3 fats in the diet to assure adequate levels of omega-3 fats so omega-3 fats can inhibit the conversion of omega-6 fats into inflammatory components [100].

The ratio of omega-6 to omega-3 fats in the American diet has increased dramatically from 1.5:1 to 16:1 (or more) because of increased consumption of wheat, foods from animals fed corn and soy (instead of grass), farmed fish (also grain-fed), soy products, and soybean oil [101]. Top sources of omega-6 fats in the American diet include chicken dishes, grain-based desserts, salad dressing, chips, pizza, breads, and fried potatoes [102].

Ideally you should get three kinds of omega-3 fats from foods: DHA (docosahexaenoic acid) and EPA (eicosapenternoic acid) from fish and seafood, and ALA (alpha linolenic acid) from plants. Our bodies can convert ALA to DHA and EPA, but only in limited amounts.

Improving omega-3 availability requires increasing omega-3 fat intake while reducing omega-6 fats from foods because these fats compete for metabolic enzymes. Our recommended eating pattern emphasizes foods high in omega-3 fats including cold-water fish (such as tuna, salmon, and mackerel), as well as other types of seafood, dark green leafy vegetables, flaxseed, walnuts, grass-fed meats, etc. We de-emphasize foods that contain primarily omega-6 fats including chicken, wheat, soy, fried foods, grain-fed animal products, etc.

Omega-3 recommendations based on American Heart Association guidelines include [103]:

- If you have not been diagnosed with coronary artery disease: eat a variety of fatty fish (see the shopping guide in Appendix A) at least twice a week and eat ALA rich foods such as walnut oil, walnuts, flaxseed, pumpkin seeds, etc.

- If you have coronary artery disease, ask your medical care provider about supplements or dietary changes to provide about 1 g of EPA and DHA per day plus ALA.

- If you are on medication to lower your triglycerides or cholesterol: ask your medical care provider about supplements or a prescription to provide 2-4 g of EPA and DHA per day plus ALA.

For more information on supplements, see "Omega-3 Fats" on page 99.

What to look for

- Eggs: organic eggs from pastured hens and 'omega-3 eggs' from hens fed flaxseed (provides ALA) or fishmeal (provides DHA) are higher in omega-3 fats. Other eggs have more omega-6 fats from corn and soy based diets.

- Dairy: look for organic dairy or products from Ireland and other locations where cows eat mostly grass, other green fodder, or silage.

- Beef: organic grass-fed and finished beef will have more omega-3 fats. Other beef will be primarily omega-6 fats because cows are fattened-up with corn, soy, and other grains in feedlots before slaughter.

- Poultry: free range and organic birds are better but are likely to be high in omega-6 fats from eating corn and soy; legs and thighs are dark meat and provide additional nutrients. Smaller 'heritage breed' birds or grass fed chickens have less fat but can be difficult to find.

- Pork: look for pasture raised and organic.

- Lamb: grass fed or pasture raised.

- Fish: fatty fish, wild fish have more omega-3 fats and are preferable to farmed fish with more omega-6 fats from corn and soy feeds.

- Processed foods with added omega-3 are not recommended for multiple reasons including small amounts of added ALA or DHA. For example: milk drinks, juice drinks, margarine, breads, sauces, pasta, etc.

Inulin

Inulin is a specific type of dietary fiber that supports beneficial gut bacteria and overall health including functions that are important for lymphedema or lipedema. Adequate inulin intake helps prevent chronic low-grade inflammation and improve immune function [104].

Not eating enough inulin can contribute to a variety of health issues including inflammation, obesity, metabolic syndrome, and type 2 diabetes. Current European diets and traditional Mediterranean diets include more inulin than the typical American diet and are associated with lower rates of obesity and diabetes.

Inulin stimulates the growth of bacteria that provide beneficial functions:

- Producing short-chain fatty acids (SCFA) including butyric acid (butyrate) that have powerful anti-inflammatory effects in the gut and throughout the body.

- Converting soy isoflavones into their more beneficial metabolite (equol).

- Helping eliminate excess estrogen via urine and feces (see "Maintaining Estrogen Regulation" on page 53). Excess estrogen, due to impaired elimination, has negative health effects on both sexes.

Helpful gut microbes produce short-chain fatty acids which are important nutrients and influence the production of hormones, which affect the whole body including [105]:

- Neurotransmitters that lift mood, increase positive emotions and reward-seeking, and support thinking, such as serotonin, dopamine, noradrenaline, and GABA. Neurotransmitters also help regulate gut motility.

- Gastrointestinal hormones that control metabolism, appetite, insulin sensitivity, blood glucose control, gut motility, and fat deposition, such as ghrelin, leptin, glucagon-like-peptide-1 (GLP-1), and peptide PYY.

- Hormones that reduce the stress response and inflammation, or promote wound healing, such as cortisol.

Inulin also helps reduce the loss of beneficial microbes during antibiotic treatment.

At least 2.5 grams of inulin per day appears to be the minimum for supporting healthy gut bacteria. Additional benefit may be seen with up to 10 grams per day. Large quantities of inulin or rapid increases in intake can cause diarrhea. If you have fructose malabsorption, NCGS, or irritable bowel syndrome (IBS) you may need to limit your inulin intake.

We do not yet have tests for inulin levels or the health of gut microbes. You can estimate your inulin intake using the data on inulin content of foods in Table 5-1 [106]. If you think you would benefit from additional inulin, try eating more inulin-containing food or taking supplements (see "Inulin Fiber" on page 100) and see if you notice any difference after three weeks.

Table 5-1: Food Sources of Inulin

Food	Inulin Grams/ Serving	Serving Size	Serving Size Ounces	Serving Size Grams	Inulin g/100 g
Banana, raw	0.5	One small (6-7")	3.6	101	0.5
Asparagus, raw	3.4	Cup	4.7	134	2.5
Asparagus, boiled	1.5	Cup	3.2	90	1.7
Chicory Root	18.7	Cup	1.6	45	41.6
Dandelion Greens, raw	6.9	Cup chopped	1.9	55	12.5
Dandelion Greens, cooked	9.6	Cup chopped	3.7	105	9.1
Garlic, raw	0.4	One clove	0.1	3	12.5
Artichoke (Globe)	5.3	One medium	4.2	120	4.4
Jerusalem Artichoke or Sunchoke	27.0	Cup of slices	5.3	150	18
Leeks, raw	5.8	Cup of slices	3.1	89	6.5
Onions, raw	0.6	One medium slice	0.5	14	4.3
Onions, cooked	2.8	Medium onion	3.3	94	3.0
Wheat Flour, baked	3.0	Cup	4.4	125	2.4

Other foods that are good sources of inulin include Belgian endive, burdock, curly endive, escarole, frisee, jicama, radicchio, red treviso, salsify, and yacon. Some manufactured foods include inulin from chicory root extract as a fat replacement.

Wheat provided 69% of the inulin in the American diet in the 1990's (the most recent study) [107]. Since then, wheat consumption is lower overall and many people eat little (low-carb diet) or no (gluten-free) wheat [108]. The inulin content of wheat may also be lower [109], and milling changes may have reduced the inulin in flour.

Fermented Foods

Fermented foods contain live bacteria that help stimulate the immune system and maintain a healthy and diverse mix of gut microbes. Some fermented foods also contain enzymes that improve digestion and short-chain fatty acids.

Kefir is especially good because it contains beneficial microbes that help correct gut dysbiosis, very little milk sugar (lactose) and no added sugars (unflavored). Kefir does not trigger lactose intolerance and may improve lactose digestion. Try kefir as a drink or a topping for cereal or berries.

Look for fermented products in the refrigerator case with other dairy or specialty foods. For example, kefir and yogurt with active cultures, sauerkraut, dill or kosher pickles, kimchi (mild or spicy), tempeh, miso, natto, etc.

Pickles (and similar products) that do not require refrigeration are 'vinegar pickles' made using vinegar brine and do not provide bacteria from fermentation.

Artificial Sweeteners

Artificial sweeteners and sugar substitutes should be avoided for several reasons:

- Non-nutritive sweeteners such as saccharin, sucralose and aspartame directly induce a propensity for obesity and glucose intolerance by changing the mix and function of the gut microbes (intestinal microbiota) in animal models [110].

- Sweeteners containing sugar alcohols such as isomalt, mannitol, sorbitol, xylitol, etc. can trigger digestive problems, especially in anyone who is sensitive to fructose or FODMAP foods.

These and other artificial sweeteners are in the list of ingredients to avoid in Appendix B.

Instead of artificial sweeteners, try using regular sugar in progressively smaller amounts. For coffee or tea, try different varieties and see if there are flavors that you can enjoy without sweetener or with less sugar. Replace nondairy creamer or coffee whiteners with unsweetened almond milk, low- or non-fat milk.

Chapter 6:

Vitamins, Minerals, and Supplements

If you have, or are at risk for, lymphedema or lipedema you are likely to benefit from vitamins, minerals, and supplements to provide nutritional factors you cannot obtain reliably, or in adequate quantities, from food sources. Your need for additional nutrients may change as you change your eating pattern, your health changes, or you get older.

Our recommendations include three categories:

1. Vitamins and Minerals everyone should consider taking daily.

2. Routine Supplements to consider taking regularly.

3. As Needed Supplements for specific needs or occasional use.

If you are at risk for lymphedema or lipedema but do not have symptoms consider:

• Vitamins and Minerals

• Routine Supplements, with the possible exception of Butcher's Broom.

Our list includes supplements that the authors or their patients have found to be beneficial. Some supplements have overlapping effects and we are not suggesting that anyone try or take all of these supplements.

Suggested doses are for an average adult. Dosages may need to be adjusted based on body weight for smaller or larger individuals. If in doubt, start with a smaller dose and increase gradually.

There is some thinking that varying supplements periodically or not taking supplements every day may have some health benefits. For example, some people take them five days a week. Certainly, you should not be upset if you miss a day.

As always, your mileage may vary, evaluate your need for each and consult your health care provider, as appropriate. Be sure to include all vitamins, minerals, supplements, and over-the-counter medications on your medication list.

Look for supplements from established brand names with third party testing seals that verify ingredients (such as USP Verified) or NSF International good manufacturing practices (GMP) certification. Check labels carefully for the quantities of active ingredients.

Vitamins and Minerals

Consider taking these vitamins and minerals routinely.

Multivitamins

Good quality multivitamins with minerals provide an easy way to ensure adequate intake of nutrients such as iodine and fluoride that are sometimes difficult to obtain from food sources.

Vitamin B-12

Many patients with lymphedema or lipedema have vitamin B12 deficiency risk factors and low B12 levels may contribute to common lymphedema symptoms such as tiredness, depression, weakness, constipation, and numbness or tingling in the hands and feet [111]. The Institute of Medicine recommends B-12 supplements for anyone over 50 or with B-12 deficiency risk factors [112].

Dosage: 500-1,000 mcg/day from sublingual spray or tablets. Injections are preferable for conditions that impair absorption such as Crohn's disease. B12 supplements can lead to acne development in a small percentage of people [113].

Vitamin D and Calcium

Vitamin D and calcium reduce inflammation, support immune system function, and may help prevent cancer, diabetes and osteoporosis. People over 50, taking antibiotics or certain other medications, are at risk for insufficiencies in these vitamins and minerals [114].

Adequate vitamin D is especially important for anyone with or at risk for lymphedema or lipedema because vitamin D helps reduce the risk of bacterial and fungal skin infections, and helps regulate inflammation. Monitoring of blood levels (25-hydroxy vitamin D test) is recommended because some individuals may need larger doses [115].

Clinical experience: Vitamin D deficiency is very common in people with lymphedema, lipedema, digestive disorders, or liver disease.

Dosage: Consider taking supplements for vitamin D (2,000 to 4,000 IU per day) and calcium. Ask your health care provider about periodically checking your serum vitamin D and calcium. If your serum vitamin D is below 75 nmol/L (30 ng/ml), you may benefit from additional vitamin D and magnesium. Some people with lipedema or lymphedema need 5,000 to 50,000 IU/day of supplemental vitamin D but high doses should be monitored for side effects.

Vitamin D can interact with certain drugs. For example, steroids such as prednisone, can impair vitamin D metabolism; weight-loss drugs such as orlistat, and cholesterol-lowering medications, such as cholestyramine, can reduce the absorption of vitamin D and other fat-soluble vitamins [116].

Calcium can interact with certain drugs. For example, calcium can decrease absorption of bisphosphonates for osteoporosis, the fluoroquinolone and tetracycline classes of antibiotics, levothyroxine, phenytoin, and tiludronate disodium. Thiazide-type diuretics can interact with calcium carbonate and vitamin D supplements, increasing the risks of hypercalcemia and hypercalciuria. Aluminum- and magnesium-containing antacids increase calcium excretion. Mineral oil and stimulant laxatives decrease calcium absorption. Glucocorticoids, such as prednisone, can cause calcium depletion [117].

Magnesium

Magnesium is an essential ion for the brain, heart, and skeletal muscles, with anti-inflammatory properties. Plant based foods containing dietary fiber are good sources of magnesium. For example nuts, seeds, dark green leafy vegetables, beans or legumes, and whole grains.

Water can be an important source of magnesium but the magnesium content of tap water and bottled waters varies widely. Bottled spring waters are mineral-deficient and provide little or no magnesium, making them less desirable than most North American tap water or mineral water as sources of magnesium but [118].

The recommended daily intake is 420 mg for men and 320 mg for women. At least 60% of North Americans do not get adequate amounts of magnesium from food including 89% of teenaged girls, 55–58% of persons aged 51–70 years, and 70–80% of individuals over 70. There is no simple test for whole body magnesium status [119].

Mild magnesium deficiency causes nonspecific symptoms such as depression, tiredness, muscle spasms, and muscle weakness. Low magnesium levels (serum magnesium below 0.7 mM) are associated with chronic inflammation, coronary artery disease, atrial fibrillations, type 2 diabetes, and hypertension. Severe deficiency can lead to cardiac arrhythmias, muscle contractions (tetany), or seizures. Magnesium supplements have shown benefit in treating migraine, depression, coronary artery disease, asthma, and other conditions [120].

Many factors contribute to magnesium deficiency including diets high in processed foods and refined grains where 80 to 90% of magnesium is lost during processing, a long term 20 –30% decrease in magnesium content of fruits and vegetables due to soil depletion, and other factors discussed below. High calcium intake (such as from supplements) can contribute to low magnesium status and vice versa because of calcium-magnesium interactions.

Magnesium inadequacy results from a combination of factors including low intake of foods containing magnesium, impaired ability to absorb magnesium in the gut, or greater than normal magnesium elimination.

Conditions that increase the risk of magnesium inadequacy include [121]:

- Advanced age: older adults have lower dietary intake of magnesium, decreased magnesium absorption, and increased magnesium excretion.

- Proton pump inhibitors and certain types of diuretics, antibiotics, antifungals, anti-cancer drugs, and other medications increase the risk of magnesium depletion [122].

- Chronic diarrhea or fat malabsorption from gastrointestinal diseases such as celiac disease, Crohn's disease, or regional enteritis.

- Resection or bypass of the small intestine, especially the ileum.

- Metabolic syndrome or Type 2 diabetes.

- Alcohol dependence or frequent alcohol consumption.

- Fatty liver disease or chronic kidney disease.

Excess magnesium from food is not a health risk. Tolerable upper intake levels for supplemental magnesium is 350 mg/day for ages 9 and up. High doses of magnesium from supplements (including multivitamins) or drugs containing magnesium—such as Epsom salts, antacids, cathartics, laxatives, and enemas—can cause diarrhea, nausea, and abdominal cramping. Elevated serum magnesium (greater than 1.1 mM) can cause vomiting, lethargy, headaches, flushing, or diminished deep tendon reflexes. Higher magnesium levels can cause somnolence, loss of deep tendon reflexes, hypotension, severe cardiac defects, coma, and death [123].

There are several ways to increase magnesium levels:

- Soaking in warm water (not hot water) with Epsom salts, Dead Sea salts, magnesium flakes, or other magnesium-based bath salts. Magnesium is absorbed through the skin and helps improve skin barrier function and hydration while reducing inflammation.

- Oral magnesium supplements are available in pills, powders, and liquid forms.

- Topical magnesium supplements such as oils, gels, sprays, etc.

- Intravenous infusion or injected magnesium supplements are sometimes used for pain control or to increase magnesium levels while bypassing the digestive tract.

Over-the-counter digestive medications containing magnesium are not helpful for increasing magnesium levels because they contain forms of magnesium that are not well absorbed. Avoid combining these medications with supplemental magnesium.

Clinical experience: Supplemental magnesium can be helpful for muscle cramps and pain in lymphedema and lipedema. Soaking affected feet in warm (not hot) water with Epsom salts helps improve skin condition. Dry feet thoroughly after soaking, especially between the toes.

Age-related subclinical magnesium deficiency may benefit from supplements even when serum magnesium levels are normal. A randomized clinical trial showed 300 mg/day of magnesium for 12 weeks had a significant positive effect on physical performance of healthy elderly women. Improvement was more evident in women with dietary magnesium intakes below the RDA [124].

Dosage: Consider taking magnesium supplements providing 250-350 mg of magnesium per day, such as oral magnesium malate, magnesium citrate or magnesium chloride. Take oral supplements with food, as directed on the package.

Check with your health care provider about potential drug interactions (see below) or if you would benefit from higher doses of supplemental magnesium based on your risk factors for magnesium inadequacy (discussed above). Higher doses can help replenish magnesium stores in those who have been deficient for some time.

Several types of medications may interact with magnesium supplements or affect magnesium levels. For example, oral bisphosphonates such as Fosamax, some antibiotics including tetracyclines, such as demeclocycline and doxycycline, as well as quinolone antibiotics, such as ciprofloxacin and levofloxacin, diuretics, and proton pump inhibitors such as Nexium and Prevacid [125]. Also certain antifungals, anti-cancer drugs, and other medications [126].

Selenium

Selenium is an essential trace mineral that helps protect against oxidative cell damage, regulate thyroid function, and support the immune system. Studies show that higher blood levels of selenium are associated with fewer cancer cases and lower death rates from cancer. Selenium deficiency contributes to certain diseases and makes the body more susceptible to illness.

Selenium enhances the effectiveness of CDT in lymphedema treatment. The low toxicity profile of selenium and its cost effectiveness are further arguments for its use in lymphedema care [127].

Clinical experience: Supplemental selenium appears to help reduce swelling and weight with both lymphedema and lipedema, even in the absence of deficiency. Consider additional selenium from a supplement or Brazil nuts if you have swelling.

Dosage: 400-600 mcg/day from a supplement OR eat a maximum of 6 Brazil nuts per day purchased shelled (about 1 ounce) or 3 nuts per day purchased unshelled.

If you have gastrointestinal disease, a history of severe infections, or have had weight loss surgery you may have difficulty absorbing selenium; ask your medical care provider about monitoring your selenium level [128].

Routine Supplements

Consider taking these supplements routinely.

Omega-3 Fats

If you have coronary artery disease, take medication to lower your triglycerides or cholesterol, or do not routinely eat fatty fish, you should consider omega-3 supplements for additional DHA/EPA.

Most omega-3 supplements are either DHA/EPA (omega-3 fats found in seafood) or ALA (the omega-3 from plants). If you are allergic to fish, shellfish, or seafood, check with your health care provider about which DHA/EPA supplements are best for you.

DHA/EPA supplement options include:

- Fish oil capsules from manufacturers who test for mercury and other toxins should not pose the same risk of contamination as fish.

- Krill oil supplements are made from crustaceans and may contain smaller amounts of DHA than fish oil capsules. Some products combine krill oil and fish oil.

- Algae or microalgae based DHA supplements are suitable for vegans.

ALA supplements are typically flaxseed oil. Large quantities can cause diarrhea.

Dosage: See "Omega-3 vs. Omega-6 Fats" on page 85 for guidelines on omega-3 intake from foods and supplements for different medical conditions.

Inulin Fiber

Inulin is a specific type of dietary fiber available from many food sources, as explained in "Inulin" on page 87. Consider supplemental inulin if you are not able to get enough inulin from food sources, especially if you are taking antibiotics or have been on antibiotics in the past month.

Inulin or fructo-oligosaccharides (FOS) supplements are available as capsules, powders, and chewable gummies. Inulin supplements may be classified as fiber supplements or prebiotics.

Dosage: 8-10 grams/day from a combination of food sources and supplements.

Inulin can cause gas, bloating or diarrhea in larger amounts or when first taking supplements. Taking smaller amounts with meals can help. Digestive conditions such as fructose malabsorption, NCGS (inulin is a FODMAP compound), or irritable bowel syndrome (IBS) may be triggered by inulin, especially if combined with high fructose foods like honey or fruits [129]. Butyrate supplements are an alternative used to treat IBS [130].

Butcher's Broom

Butcher's broom, a powdered extract derived from the Ruscus aculeatus plant, increases fluid movement within lymph vessels by binding as an agonist to alpha-adrenergic receptors on lymph cells. Butcher's broom may decrease lymphedema by enhancing smooth muscle inducement of lymphatic flow and thereby increasing lymphatic drainage. Ruscogenins from this plant are reportedly effective for preventing or treating chronic venous insufficiency. Butcher's broom for lymphatic flow combined with selenium for anti-inflammatory properties are useful in treating lipedema and lipolymphedema [131].

Clinical experience: Lymphedema and lipedema patients report good results with Butcher's broom. In a published case, a 67-year-old woman with stage II lipedema and lipolymphedema was able to maintain a volume reduction of 1,262 ml per leg on a combination of Butcher's broom, selenium and CDT [**132**].

Dosage: 1 gm/day.

Butcher's broom is generally regarded as safe [**133**] but there is one report of toxicity in a patient with diabetes [**134**].

L-Arginine

L-arginine supplements appear to help with lymphedema and lipedema by increasing nitric oxide availability and improving lymphatic vascular integrity.

L-arginine supplements raise plasma levels briefly. Consider multiple doses per day, time-release l-arginine supplements, or L-citrulline supplements. L-Citrulline is converted to l-arginine by the kidneys, providing a longer acting source of arginine.

Clinical experience: L-arginine is beneficial for lymphedema and lipedema. For example, one 84-year-old overweight woman with lipedema who was not able to change her eating pattern lost 10 pounds in the first month on l-arginine and has maintained her lower weight for two years.

Dosage: 9 g/day as three divided doses. Dosage for congestive heart failure range from 6-20 grams per day, as three divided doses. L-arginine may interact with medications for diabetes, high blood pressure, anticoagulant medication (aspirin, clopidogrel (Plavix), dalteparin (Fragmin), enoxaparin (Lovenox), heparin, ticlopidine (Ticlid), warfarin (Coumadin), etc.), medications to increase blood flow to the heart (nitroglycerin (Nitro-Bid, Nitro-Dur, Nitrostat) or isosorbide (Imdur, Isordil, Sorbitrate), Sildenafil (Viagra), or diuretics [**135**]. Check with your medical care provider before taking this supplement, especially if you are taking these types of medications.

Curcumin or Turmeric

Curcumin is a potent anti-inflammatory and antioxidant with multiple health benefits found in turmeric and certain other spices. We did not find research specific to lymphedema or lipedema but curcumin has been shown to reduce edema related to diabetes [136].

Dosage: 500 to 2,000 mg per day. Look for a supplement with curcumin and black pepper extract (piperine) that aids in the absorption of curcumin in the GI tract. Start with a low dose and build up gradually to avoid cramping or diarrhea. Larger doses may be recommended to reduce the risk of cancer recurrence.

If you have gallstones, a bile duct obstruction, or GERD, curcumin may make your condition worse. Taking turmeric might slow blood clotting. Curcumin might decrease blood sugar in people with diabetes. Curcumin can affect how some drugs are absorbed [137]. Check with your health care provider before starting this supplement.

As Needed Supplements

Consider taking these supplements on an as-needed basis, for increased swelling or other issues (see the information below).

Flavonoids

Flavonoids or bioflavonoids are a class of chemical compounds from plant sources that includes isoflavones, flavones, and coumestans. Benzopyrones such as coumarin are flavonoids.

Flavonoids have many health benefits, as discussed above. Our recommended eating pattern emphasizes food sources of flavonoids, except for soy isoflavones.

Most supplements contain flavonoids from non-food plants such as butcher's broom, horse chestnut, or pine bark, or concentrated extracts from foods like turmeric.

Diosmin is a type of flavonoid made from chemically modified hesperidin. Diosmin is available in the US as nonprescription supplements or a prescription-only medical food (Vasculera or diosmiplex) indicated for the clinical dietary management of the metabolic processes of chronic venous insufficiency. Outside the US, diosmin may be a prescription medication (Daflon or other trade names) or a supplement.

Research on treating lymphedema with flavonoids (other than coumarin, which can cause liver damage) has not shown consistent effectiveness [138]. Research on flavonoids for lipedema focused on specific supplements, such as butcher's broom.

Supplements contain larger amounts of flavonoids than found in foods. Although supplements are natural, they are not automatically safe at all doses. Toxicity issues and drug interactions should be considered. Flavonoid supplements may affect trace element, folate, and vitamin C status and can affect thyroid function by interfering with iodine uptake [139].

Clinical experience: Bioflavonoids can be helpful for lymphedema and lipedema.

Dosage: Consider taking one of these supplements at a time, on a rotating basis:

- Citrus Bioflavonoids (Rutin, Diosmin, Hesperidin)
  Lymphedema: 500 mg twice/day with food
  Lipedema: start 500 mg twice/day and increase to 1,500 mg twice/day

- Horse Chestnut Seed Extract: 250 mg twice/day with food

- Pycnogenol (pine bark extract): 200 mg/day

Mycelium-Ganoderma Lucidum

Ganoderma Lucidum (also known as Ling-Zhi or Reishi) is a medicinal mushroom used in traditional Chinese medicine with a broad range of pharmacological properties including anti-inflammatory effects. Supplements containing triterpenes and polysaccharides extracted from Ganoderma Lucidum reduce fat cell growth and fat storage while stimulating glucose uptake [140].

Clinical experience: Beneficial for lymphedema and lipedema.

Dosage: 2 800 mg tablets 2-3 times/day.

Calcium-D-Glucarate

Glucaric acid helps the body excrete excess hormones (such as estrogen) instead of reabsorbing them, by inhibiting beta-glucuronidase activity. Fruits and vegetables especially oranges, apples, grapefruits, and cruciferous vegetables contain glucaric acid. If you are not eating these foods regularly, you may benefit from supplemental calcium-D-glucarate.

Calcium-D-glucarate is the calcium salt of D-glucaric acid. Calcium-D-glucarate supplements may help increase estrogen elimination and improve weight and lipid management in some women. There are no known drug interactions with calcium-D-glucarate [141].

Dosage: 3,000 mg/day, take supplements as directed.

Systemic Enzymes

Systemic enzyme supplements contain proteolytic enzymes packaged in an enteric-coated pill. For example, Wobenzym, Phlogenzym, Vitalzyme, etc. Unlike digestive enzyme supplements, systemic enzymes should be taken between meals. Many of these enzymes come from foods included in our recommended eating pattern, such as papaya, pineapple, mangoes, kiwi fruit, and grapes.

Systemic enzymes can help reduce inflammation and edema and speed healing following surgery or injury. Some research shows positive results for lymphedema (for example [142]); we did not find any research on lipedema.

Clinical experience: Some patients benefit from taking systemic enzymes for a few days to speed recovery from an injury or to help reduce fibrosis.

Dosage: Take as directed on the supplement package. Take either systemic enzymes or bromelain, not both.

Pineapple/Bromelain Enzyme

Bromelain enzyme in pineapple or available in supplement form has anti-inflammatory properties and may help reduce swelling. Pineapple is often recommended for lymphedema but there is little research showing effectiveness in reducing swelling and no research specific to lymphedema. Bromelain can affect the metabolism of certain antibiotics and can slow blood clotting [143].

Dosage: eat modest amounts of fresh pineapple between meals or take bromelain supplements as directed. Take either bromelain or systemic enzymes, not both.

DHEA

DHEA (dehydroepiandrosterone) is a hormone with a wide variety of neurological and biological functions including supporting estrogen synthesis in women of all ages. Circulating DHEA levels change with age, peaking in the mid-20's and declining to a low around 65-70, the age at which the frequency of age-related illnesses increases [144].

Clinical experience: Consider DHEA supplementation if you are taking cortisone or other steroids, or have signs of adrenal insufficiency (chronic fatigue, loss of appetite, muscle wasting, etc.). Ask your health care provider about testing DHEA levels before deciding about supplementation.

Dosage: 25 mg/day for women, 50 mg/day for men.

Chapter **7**:

Changing Eating Patterns

Changing your eating pattern takes a combination of four elements as explained below:

- Will or motivation to make and sustain change.

- Skills for building new habits, such as a new eating pattern.

- Acceptance of responsibility for behaviors you control (progress toward your goals); while letting go of things you that are not under your control and acknowledging that your condition may vary, even with the best possible care.

- Experimentation to learn what works for your body.

- Overcoming emotional issues related to eating or food choices.

Will

If you are already convinced and ready to change your eating pattern, skip to "Write Down Your Reasons" on page 112. If you are not sure, use these tools to help you decide what changes, if any, you want to make at this time.

Ability to change is like a muscle, it gets stronger with use but can become strained and cramped if you push too hard. Pace your changes to avoid becoming overloaded and frustrated.

You may have more than one behavior you would like to change. These changes may relate to self-care, stress, exercise, etc. Many people find it easier to focus on one behavior change at a time, especially for changes that involve learning new skills. Others prefer to make related changes together, like healthier eating and exercising.

Practice each new behavior long enough to create habits before starting your next change. New eating habits go through two stages: 1) eating according to a set of rules (external knowledge), 2) learning the rules and skills well enough to internalize them and follow them automatically (internal knowledge). You can make these changes at your own pace. Some people continue charting after they have internalized their new eating pattern.

Prioritizing what to change is up to you, in consultation with your health care providers. In general, we suggest that if you have lymphedema or lipedema that affects your feet, effective skin care should be your top priority, followed by improving eating patterns and other self-care skills. If your feet are not affected, you may want to start with nutrition.

Changing your eating pattern can overlap with treatment (CDT) for lymphedema or lipedema. If you are depressed (see "Depression" on page 123), you may benefit from starting therapy for depression before changing your eating pattern.

Objectives and Goals

In talking about change, we make a distinction between objectives and goals. Although this seems like a small difference now, it can become important later.

The way we use these terms:

- Objectives are your reasons for changing, your expected benefits, how changes will improve your life

- Goals are actions under your control that should help you meet your objectives. For example, following a new eating pattern 5 days this week, getting 30 minutes of exercise every day, etc.

Ideally, meeting your goals will accomplish your objectives but this may not always be the case for reasons we cannot predict or control.

Decision Balance

If you are undecided about changing your eating pattern, take some time to think through your options. You may want to change what you eat, make other changes, or continue on your current course without changes.

Decision balance analysis will help you organize your thoughts, evaluate your options, and make an informed decision [145].

People change when the motivation for a new behavior (the change) becomes greater than the motivation for keeping their current pattern (maintaining the status quo). Writing down the advantages and disadvantages of each alternative will help you organize your thoughts, identify all the factors you want to consider, and evaluate your alternatives systematically.

To evaluate decision balance:

- Frame your question as two alternatives. Usually these are changing or maintaining but you can also use this technique to decide between changes.

- Make two charts, one for each alternative, with columns for the advantages and disadvantages of each alternative. See the sidebar Decision Balance Example on page 110.

- Fill in the advantages and disadvantages for each alternative.

- Compare charts to be sure that all the factors you care about are included for each alternative.

- Optionally, drill deeper into each factor by asking why or how.

If you are big and the idea of changing to a smaller size makes you uncomfortable or anxious, consider talking to a mental health professional about these feelings.

Decision Balance Example	
Changing: New Eating Pattern	
Advantages	**Disadvantages**
☐ I'll improve my health	☐ It's hard work
☐ I'll have more energy	☐ I'll have to give up sweets and treats
☐ I'll look better	☐ I may feel extra hungry
	☐ I may feel stressed
Maintaining: Current Eating Pattern	
Advantages	**Disadvantages**
☐ It is easy	☐ I won't get healthier
☐ I can eat favorite foods	☐ I might end up gaining weight
☐ I can relieve stress by snacking	☐ I might get sick and face large doctor's bills

Imaging or Visualizing Alternatives

Picturing yourself looking or acting in certain ways is another tool for evaluating alternatives and building motivation. Positive imaging involves seeing yourself making progress towards your goals or having reached them. How will you look and act? What will you be doing? How will your life be different? Negative imaging reflects your fears and situations you would like to avoid by making changes [146].

The process is similar to decision balance analysis but using images:

- Frame your question as two alternatives. Usually these are changing or maintaining but you can also use this technique to decide between changes.

- Collect or draw two sets of pictures, one for each alternative, showing things you might do, how you might look, other things that you care about for each alternative.

- Add additional images showing changes in your daily life and routine for each alternative. What does a meal look like? Where do you shop? What is a typical day?

If you prefer other media, try:

- Visualizing yourself as you go through your daily routine for each alternative. What are the differences and how do they feel?

- Writing a story about a day in your future life for each scenario. What will your routine include?

- Identifying a role model for each alternative based on someone you know personally, someone you have heard about, or a character from a movie or novel; think or write about what they would do, if they were in your position. Feel free to use other conditions or physical challenge in place of lymphedema or lipedema.

- Selecting music that represents each option or has appropriate lyrics. What would be on your playlist?

- Sketching graphs of factors that are important to you and how these quantities change over time in each scenario. Consider the rate of change as shown by the slope of the graph.

Start Keeping Records

Track your weight, meals, and mood based on the instructions in "Foods and Moods" on page 224 for a few weeks. Women who are menstruating will need at least five weeks of data to be able to compare the same days of their menstrual cycle.

Weight changes are common in women with lipedema. Some women vary several pounds during the day as well as changing from one day to the next.

Look at the data and the trend:

- What were your mood and energy levels and how are they changing?

- How does your current eating pattern compare to our recommendations?

- How many times a day are you eating?

- What is the overall trend for your weight? How quickly is it changing?

- Are you eating for emotional reasons? See "Overcoming Emotional Issues" on page 123 for suggestions or consult a licensed mental health professional.

- If you drink alcohol and are concerned that you might have trouble stopping, ask your health care provider about helpful options.

For a better understanding of your current eating pattern, and how you might benefit from changing, try keeping a food diary (see "Food Diary" on page 226). A Basic Food Diary will give you a better idea of what you are eating. Counting carbohydrates or doing nutritional analysis will show how your energy intake (calories consumed from food) compares to your energy expenditure (calories used at rest and in activities) and what benefits you might expect from changing your eating pattern.

Note: Check with your health care provider if your weight changes rapidly and the change (up or down) is not consistent with your eating habits and activities. Unexpected weight change can be a symptom of many health issues.

Write Down Your Reasons

When you have decided what change you want, write down your thoughts so you can organize and clarify your ideas. Save your reasons to review them later to reinforce your motivation, or revise your thinking based on new information.

You may find it helpful to set specific objectives and goals:

- Objectives: should reflect your reasons for changing, the benefits you expect, and how these changes will improve your life

- Goals: activities you control that will help meet your objectives. For example, following a new eating pattern 5 days this week, getting more exercise, etc.

Ideally meeting your goals will accomplish your objectives. However, we know that these conditions can be unpredictable and progress towards your objectives may vary for many reasons.

It Takes **Your** Village

If you eat with others regularly (family, friends, roommates, coworkers, etc.), changing your eating pattern may have implications for what group members eat, where you eat (if you go out), and your relationship with the group. Consider these changes as part of your decision process and prepare to discuss or negotiate changes with the group. Hopefully you will be able to enlist their support. They may even join you in healthier eating, at least for a trial period.

You may have several groups to consider including your significant other, relatives, people you live with, coworkers, social groups that involve eating, etc. Focus on the groups where you share more than one meal each week.

Start by filling out Decision Balance charts from the viewpoint of group members, not yourself. Based on what you know about group members:

• What would they see as the advantages and disadvantages of the status quo?

• What advantages and disadvantages would they experience if they changed to your new eating plan along with you? Are there any reasons they could not make this change, at least for the meals you share?

• If you changed to a new eating plan, but they continued their current eating pattern unchanged, what would be the advantages and disadvantages for them? What are the practical implications of this split?

If you think your group may not be willing to change to your new eating plan, make Decision Balance charts from your viewpoint for other options:

• If you change to your new eating plan and your group continues their current eating plan, what are the advantages and disadvantages for you? What are the practical implications?

• Optionally, consider what you might do if you leave this group and go on your own or change to a different group, and the advantages and disadvantages.

After you have organized your thoughts, you can discuss or negotiate this change with members of your groups. Think about what you are asking them to do or change, how they may benefit from this change, and your alternatives if you are not able to reach agreement.

Things you may want to cover include:

- Your reasons for changing your eating pattern including what you hope to accomplish (your objectives) and key steps in the process (your goals).

- An overview of your new eating pattern and key areas where it will be different, illustrated with some specific menu examples.

- Asking them to help you by supporting your change, if appropriate. (The next section includes more detail on how they can help.)

- Ask if they are interesting in changing their eating pattern and if they are interested, describe what you see as the advantages and disadvantages for them. Ask their views on the factors you identified and see what other factors they suggest.

- Discuss how their changing to your new eating pattern, or not changing, will affect you in terms of the advantages and disadvantages. Check your perceptions with them, find out how they see these issues, and ask about other factors or concerns.

If you are still not sure if you want to change your eating pattern, or you have identified barriers to changing, check with your health care provider and see if they can suggest additional resources.

Skills

Building new habits can involve two types of skills: habit-building skills, like the ones described below, and skills required for implementing the new habit, such as shopping and food preparation.

This section provides habit-building skills based on research into behavior change in general and specific strategies for changing eating patterns.

Make Specific Plans

Discuss your goals and options with friends, family, and health care providers who can provide specific information and supportive feedback.

Simple keys for successful change:

* Make very specific plans: when will you start? What do you need first? What is the next step?

* Write down your plans. It may be old school but it does increase commitment.

* Tell your friends what you are doing, explain why you are doing it, and ask them to support your change. Do this face-to-face, if possible.

Create Reinforcements

Reinforcement can support and maintain motivation by rewarding desired behavior changes or discouraging un-desired behaviors. Reinforcements are based on progress toward or reaching your goals, not your objectives. You are only accountable for behaviors under your control.

Positive reinforcement rewards and strengthens ("reinforces") new activities by providing something desirable. Positive reinforcements are pleasurable events, experiences, gifts, actions, etc. earned by making changes that bring you closer to your goals.

Negative reinforcement also rewards and strengthens ("reinforces") new behaviors. Negative reinforcement occurs when a desired behavior removes or avoids something unpleasant, like parental nagging.

Punishment, or negative consequences, can also support change by making failure to reach a goal more unpleasant. For example, agreeing to donate money to an organization you dislike or being required to do something constructive but not especially pleasant.

In general, positive and negative reinforcement are more effective for building skills than punishment or negative consequences. In addition, punishment or negative consequences create negative feelings and no one likes feeling bad. Using reinforcements is a matter of personal preference. If you have changed your behavior successfully in the past, continue to use the tools that work for you.

Many people find it helpful to share reinforcement plans with their friends. This has several advantages:

- Friends can help you change by creating, arranging, or providing rewards.

- Sharing progress with your friends provide another level of accountability.

- Enjoying reward activities together can strengthen relationships.

- Those who enjoy competing can arrange contests with their friends.

Here are some suggestions for this process:

- Write down the conditions for each goal or intermediate reward.

- Select rewards that are meaningful to you and your support group, and consistent with your goals. Online services can help; for example, www.stickk.com will track positive or negative financial commitments.

- Make your progress visible by sharing your records with your group or online where everyone can see them.

- Build a feeling of momentum by creating your chart with some weeks completed, giving yourself credit for what you have done already.

- Plan a series of reinforcement events at different times including 70% completed and (of course) 100%. The 70% mark is an important motivational point, showing you are close to your goal.

- Mark reward events on your future records so you see your progress towards your next reward every day.

Build Support

Try these strategies for increasing support from family, friends, and colleagues [147]:

- Make a list of supportive people in your life and keep your list up-to-date. You will feel better knowing that you have a support network and working from a list can make it easier to get assistance when you need it.

- Look for opportunities to help others in your network; build-up your favor bank whenever you can.

- Confide in people you trust about changes you are making, how you are feeling, and how you see things.

- When you need help, ask clearly for assistance and be specific about what people can do to help you.

- Grow your network by volunteering, joining clubs, taking classes, and interacting with people in other settings.

Start Smaller

Consider three scenarios for changing your eating pattern:

- **Big Bang**: eat only foods on the Eat Primarily list for the first two weeks; add foods from the Eat Occasionally list during weeks 3-6.

- **Weekend Warrior**: follow our recommended eating pattern on weekends; optionally prepare enough food on the weekend to eat recommended foods for an additional day or two.

- **Begin with Breakfast**: focus on eating a healthy breakfast (based on our recommendations and including kefir or yogurt) every day and making better choices at other meals.

Most books focus on the Big Bang option for a number of reasons, including the desire to show dramatic results. A complete change may be the best approach for some people and does has benefits in terms of changing tastes and the mix of gut microbes.

However, if you are not ready or able to make such a drastic change, one of these other scenarios will provide benefits and start you on the process of changing. Health improvements will take longer because you may be changing less than half your meals (as shown in Table 7-1: Scenario vs. Impact page 118) but any change may be better for your health than your current eating pattern.

Table 7-1: Scenario vs. Impact

Scenario	Changed Meals
Big Bang	100% (21)
Weekend Warrior	29-57% (6-12)
Begin with Breakfast	33% (7)

Consider a gradual transition if you have skills gaps or learning curve issues, as explained below.

Keep in mind:

- Small improvements in food choices are better than no improvements; your eating pattern does not have to be perfect to be better.

- Guidelines for food sensitivities are the only strict rules. If you have food allergies (shellfish, peanuts, etc.), celiac disease, or other conditions triggered by specific foods, you risk misery or harm from eating forbidden foods.

Mind the Gaps

As you start to make changes, you may discover gaps in your knowledge, skills, or other resources. This is normal and healthy. Finding and filling these gaps is an important part of the change process.

Feeling that your skills are not adequate can be a source of stress. Learning and practicing to increase skills reduces stress and allows you to face formerly stressful situations without triggering a physiological stress response.

If you can anticipate where you may have gaps, you are less likely to become discouraged or frustrated. Use the checklist in the Potential Skills Issues sidebar to prioritize areas where you have skill gaps [148].

Planning and visualization can help you anticipate some issues but there is no substitute for actually doing something to increase your knowledge. Accelerate this process with a little help from your friends: find someone who eats the way you would like to and shadow them as they shop and prepare food.

Potential Skills Issues		
Priority	**Skills Issue**	**Resources**
	Lack general nutrition knowledge	Start with this book, especially Chapter 4 and Chapter 5; see also the books in Appendix E
	Prefer unhealthy foods	See "Changing Your Tastes" on page 204 and "Eat This/Not That" on page 207
	Trouble obtaining healthy foods	See Chapter 11 and ask your support network for suggestions
	Food preparation or cooking skills	See Chapter 10, Chapter 11, and ask your support network to show you
	Eating well away from home	See Chapter 11 and ask your support network for suggestions
	Changing emotional eating behaviors	See "Overcoming Emotional Issues" on page 123; consult a mental health professional
	Planning healthy meals and menus	See Chapter 8 and ask your support network for examples
	Making time for cooking	See Chapter 8 and ask your support network how they make time to cook
	Mindful eating and savoring	See "Meditation or Mindfulness" on page 122 and the resoues in Appendix E

Climb the Learning Curve

Another important part of developing new skills is the "learning curve." In manufacturing, the learning curve shows that efficiency improves with experience. In terms of food-related activities (and self-care in general), it means that the amount of time, energy, and attention required for a task becomes smaller over time. In other words, you get better and faster with practice. Tasks that require thinking and rereading the instructions at first become easier and more automatic.

Review Once a Week

Set a regular time each week—such as Sunday morning or evening—to review your records and see how you are doing and what you can improve.

Ask yourself these questions and make notes on your answers:

- What are three good things that happened in my life last week?

- What worked well in terms of eating, activities, energy, and mood?

- What would I like to have been different and what can I learn from this?

- Where can I make improvements and what should I do differently next week?

Maintenance Phase Motivation

The work of changing is not over when you reach your goal of 6-8 weeks and have created new habits. Reaching your goal is a milestone you should celebrate. It also marks the beginning of a longer phase that is more difficult for some people: maintenance.

Many people struggle with maintenance because they have not thought about it or prepared for it. Here are some suggestions to help you avoid this trap:

- Plan to keep some records on an ongoing basis. As a minimum, track your weight daily, and swelling once a week.

- Continue to review your records once a week as described above. If you spot any issues, start keeping a food diary and problem solving.

- Many people find longer-term reinforcements helpful. If these work for you, use them (see "Create Reinforcements" on page 115).

Dealing with Exceptions

Things happen and you eat a few things (or a bunch of things) that we recommend avoiding. This is not the end of the world or even a big deal.

What is important is what you do next:

- Use your meditation or mindfulness skills (see "Meditation or Mindfulness" on page 122) to calm yourself and accept what has happened.

- Resolve to get back on track as soon as you can.

- Avoid triggering emotional eating behaviors (see "Overcoming Emotional Issues" on page 123) or giving in to the 'what-the-hell effect' and eating everything in reach.

- Problem solve the reasons why this happened to see what you can learn and how you can avoid these issues in the future.

Starting Over

If you find yourself far, far away from our recommended eating pattern for any reason, start the change process over from the beginning and get back on track. The process will be easier because you do not have as many new skills to learn.

Acceptance

"Make the best use of what is in your power, and take the rest as it happens." [149]

Enhance change and long-term happiness by accepting responsibility for choices and actions that you can control while accepting that lymphedema, lipedema, and related medical conditions may vary no matter what you do.

Reward Behaviors, Learn from Results

Reward yourself for successfully reaching your goals in terms of making changes in what you do or eat. If these changes did not produce the results you had hoped for (your objectives), view this as an opportunity for learning (see "Experimentation" on page 122). Avoid the temptation to feel responsible for, or guilty about, results you cannot control and involve factors we cannot measure or understand.

Meditation or Mindfulness

Having a daily meditation practice can help you support and reinforce acceptance, balance pressures, and maintain perspective in the face of stress.

There are many options including:

- Moving meditation in yoga, qi gong, tai chi, walking meditation, etc.

- Contemplative practices like Zen meditation, mindfulness meditation, transcendental meditation, etc.

- Religious contemplation or prayer.

- Structured worry time and other thinking skills; see Chapter 16 of **Overcoming the Emotional Challenges of Lymphedema** (Lymph Notes, 2005).

Exercise or any physical activity that requires focused attention can also be beneficial. For example, dancing, gardening, and even house cleaning if done mindfully.

For more information, see Mindfulness in Appendix E: Resources.

Experimentation

There are many aspects of nutrition where individual responses vary for a variety of reasons. For example, soy can be metabolized to create different compounds depending on your genes and mix of gut bacteria. Soy metabolites can affect hormone levels differently depending on the quantity eaten.

Experimenting will help you find what foods work best for your body. Use your records (see "Foods and Moods" on page 224) to track your experiments and results in terms of energy and mood, bowel habits, weight, and other factors. It may be harder to identify changes (and take longer) if your weight varies frequently or changes during your menstrual cycle.

Try one experiment at a time. Do not start an experiment during times of medication changes, other health events, or exceptional stress.

Do not try (unless directed by a health care professional):

- Foods where you have serious allergies.

- Known triggers for digestive issues such as gluten for celiac disease or foods that trigger IBS or other intestinal conditions.

There are two types of experiments: food elimination and food trials.

Food elimination experiments look at the effect of not eating a certain food or substituting one food for another:

- Start with a baseline period during which you eat the food as usual.
- Stop or replace the food and see what the effects are over several days.
- Optionally, try reintroducing the food if the effects are not clear.

For example, how will substituting an orange (high in flavonoids) for an apple (high in fructose) at lunchtime affect your weight?

If you have been eating only foods on the Eat Primarily list and want to try adding other favorite foods, test foods on the Eat in Limited Quantities list before trying foods from the Eat Rarely or Never list.

Food trial experiments look at introducing a new food:

- Start with a small quantity of the food you want to try on one day.
- See how your body responds over a few days.
- Gradually increase the quantity or frequency if you are pleased with your response.

Overcoming Emotional Issues

Emotions are frequently a factor in eating habits and can be a barrier to changing to a healthier eating pattern. Your Foods and Moods records may show that you sometimes eat for emotional reasons or you may recognize some of these issues.

Depression

Feeling sad and sorry for oneself at times is perfectly natural. Being discouraged about dealing with a chronic condition like lymphedema or lipedema is normal but sometimes feelings of sadness stop being mild, temporary, or occasional and turn into depression.

Depression Warning Signs

☐ Wanting to die, talking about suicide, suicide plans, or suicide attempts

☐ Feeling sad, anxious or "empty" most of the day for two weeks or longer

☐ Hopelessness or pessimism

☐ Feelings of guilt, worthlessness, or helplessness

☐ Irritability, restlessness, or agitation

☐ Loss of interest in activities or hobbies that used to be pleasurable

☐ Fatigue or decreased energy

☐ Trouble concentrating, remembering details, or making decisions

☐ Trouble getting to sleep or staying asleep, waking too early, or sleeping too much

☐ Overeating or loss of appetite

☐ Persistent aches or pains, headaches, cramps or digestive problems that do not ease with treatment

If you are thinking of harming yourself, contact your health care provider immediately and take emergency action to remain safe.

Depression is a much more serious problem than brief normal sadness. Untreated depression impairs quality of life and may interfere with immune system functioning.

Review the warning signs for depression in the sidebar above. If you think you may have a clinical depression, seek help. Very effective treatments are available including specific techniques like cognitive-behavioral therapy and antidepressant medication. Talk to a licensed mental health professional. Thousands of people with depression have gotten better.

Unhealthy Patterns

Certain patterns of eating are unhealthy. Any of these eating patterns can interfere with good self-care for lymphedema or lipedema. They also interfere with overcoming the emotional challenges of these conditions because they worsen depression, lower self-esteem, and can disrupt interpersonal relationships.

Here are some warning signs of possible unhealthy eating patterns.

Ask yourself these three questions:

1. Repeatedly (not just occasionally) do you eat an unusually large amount of food in a short amount of time?

2. Do you feel out of control when you eat?

3. Do you try to prevent weight gain by making yourself throw up, by taking laxatives or diuretics, by alternating bingeing with eating too little or fasting, and/or by excessive exercising?

If you said yes to all three questions, it is possible that you have bulimia. Even if you are not overweight, this eating pattern can be terribly damaging to your health.

If you said yes to the first two questions, it is possible that you have binge eating disorder. During a binge, you may eat unusually quickly, eat despite not being hungry and/or eat until you feel physically uncomfortable. You feel out of control while eating and may feel disgusted, embarrassed, depressed, or guilty during or after binges. Binge eating is often associated with obesity.

Coping Suggestions

Notice how, when, where, and how much you eat.

Notice how you feel before, during, and after eating.

Consider seeing a mental health professional experienced in successful treatment of eating disorders. See Eating Disorders in Appendix E: Resources.

People with eating disorders often base their entire self-esteem on their weight or body shape. Eating becomes associated with conflict, guilt, shame, and struggle. The purpose of eating—nourishing and maintaining the body's health—gets lost.

Under-Eating

If your food diary shows that you are not eating adequate calories, perhaps you have another type of eating disorder. People with anorexia nervosa have a distorted body image that causes them to see themselves as fat, overweight, or imperfect even when they are normal weight or thin. They may refuse to eat, exercise compulsively, or develop unusual habits like refusing to eat while others are watching. Depression and anxiety are more common in people with eating disorders.

Physical problems associated with anorexia include anemia, constipation, osteoporosis, even damage to the heart and brain. Individuals with anorexia have a mortality rate 18 times higher than normal [**150**].

If eating behaviors are having a destructive impact on your functioning or self-image, see a mental health professional experienced in treating eating disorders.

Boredom

If you eat because you are bored [**151**]:

- Find other ways to alleviate boredom such as listening to music, talk shows, podcasts, or audio books.

- Arrange to do monotonous activities in places where you do not have easy access to food, to avoid the temptation.

- Arrange non-food rewards for completing mundane tasks.

- Fill your empty time with more interesting activities: new hobbies, groups, courses, volunteer work, etc.

- Get out with other people when you are feeling lonely and interact with them: take a walk, visit a library or bookstore, etc.

- Post a list of alternative activities where you will see it when you reach for a snack to remind you of your options. For example, on the refrigerator door.

Comfort Foods

Foods can be comforting for different reasons:

- Sugar and fat trigger reward centers in the brain and, during times of stress, slow the release of stress hormones, which helps reduce our physical stress reaction.

- Foods associated with childhood or family can provide emotional comfort by evoking feelings or memories of happiness and safety.

- Physical sensations of eating or drinking be comforting. For example, a baby can be soothed by sucking on a pacifier.

- Sharing food or drink is part of many religious ceremonies and celebrations.

- Many people have specific comfort foods, which they believe will rapidly lift them out of a negative mood.

- Preparing food for others, or having food prepared for you, is an important element in caring relationships.

Eating for comfort can produce conflicting feelings. For example, if you eat candy because you are upset, you may feel comforted initially and then feel guilty or angry with yourself for having eaten candy.

One of the challenges of changing to a new eating pattern is developing insight into your personal versions of comfort food and creating new patterns consistent with your health goals.

You may find it useful to think about various parts separately:

- What are healthy ways that I can comfort myself or lift my mood?

- What traditional or childhood foods have meaning for me? If they are not consistent with my current eating pattern, can I have small amounts or change the recipe to use healthy ingredients?

- Can I care for family and friends by providing foods that combine my eating pattern and their tastes?

- How can I explain to family and friends what I like to eat now, what I absolutely cannot eat, and what I can only have in tiny amounts?

Cravings

Combat cravings and emotional eating by pausing for a minute and using this mindfulness technique to change your thinking from habitual and self-critical emotional thinking to a calmer and more self-aware state of mind [152]:

1. Breathe in slowly through your nose, noticing the sensations of the air—perhaps its coolness as it enters your nostrils or the scent of the room. Focus on awareness of your breathing; the specifics of what you notice are not important.

2. Purse your lips and breathe out slowly, as if you were breathing through a straw. Once again, pay attention to the actual sensation of breathing, and slowing down your breathing rate.

3. Take four to eight of these mindful in-and-out breaths.

4. Return to the moment. Notice how you feel, perhaps you feel more relaxed, maybe the colors seem more vibrant, maybe your nose itches. All that matters is that you are paying attention to the here and now.

5. Focus on more reasonable self-talk, if you are still craving food. You may be more interested in other things by now. Mindfulness trains the brain to identify less with how you feel and more with the part of you that is self-aware, a witness to how you are feeling, and able to take a big picture view of what you want overall.

If you judge yourself harshly, you are more likely to feel bad and trigger emotional eating—eating to make yourself feel better. When you are gentle and compassionate with yourself to start with—mindfulness cultivates gentle compassion—you create new thinking patterns about eating and food.

Food Pushers and Sabotage

People may encourage you to eat more than you want, or to eat foods you know you should avoid. Frequently this is because they are eating in an unhealthy way and would like you to join them. Both healthy and unhealthy eating can be contagious [153].

Try these strategies:

- Tell people about your resolve to change your eating pattern in order to improve your health and ask them to support you in your efforts.

- If the occasion is a big deal (and the food is one you can eat safely) give the impression of indulging and push your plate aside after a bite or two.

- Say it looks fabulous but you could not eat another bite after the delicious meal and ask for a piece to take home for the next day (which you are not obligated to eat).

Sometimes a person who knows you are changing your eating pattern will push you to eat excessively or to eat foods you are avoiding. This sabotage can be well-intended or have other motives, and may be more about the other person than about you.

Consider these questions:

- Does this person realize they are pushing against the changes you want to make? Sometimes people offer food without thinking or do not understand which foods you are avoiding.

- Could this person feel threatened by the changes you are making or worried that your changes will change the dynamic of your relationship?

- Do they envy your ability to make changes, feel inferior or jealous?

- Are they resistant to any change, even if you are the one who is changing?

You can choose how to handle the situation:

- If someone important to you genuinely wants you to fail, confront him or her and try to negotiate a solution.

- Avoid or ignore anyone who wants you to fail but is not important to you.

- Reassure someone who feels threatened by your changes.

- Deal with well-intended or unconscious sabotage by calmly explaining how you need their help in changing and what they can do that would be most helpful for you.

Deal with Conflicts

Interpersonal relationships are especially important because stress from relationship conflicts can contribute to weight gain through increased appetite [154]. If you feel stressed by conflict in a relationship, it is important for your health to resolve this conflict–if possible–or strive to accept that you cannot change the relationship (see "Acceptance" on page 121).

While trying to resolve conflicts, it may help to [155]:

- Express yourself directly, tactfully and calmly.

- Describe your needs and feeling with statements that begin with I, followed by a request for change or action, and support for your request.

- Avoid complaining, whining, or accusations.

If necessary, seek help from your support network or a mental health professional.

Chapter 8

Meal Plans and Menus

This chapter includes example meal plans, tips for meal planning, suggested foods for different eating occasions, and transition aids for moving away from bread, pasta, and meats.

Example Meal Plans

Three meal plans:

- Recommended meal plan using the recipes provided in the next chapter.

- Actual meals from Emily Iker, our lymphedema role model.

- Actual meals from Linda-Anne Kahn, our lipedema role model.

Recommended Meal Plan

Table 8-1 on page 133 is a recommended meal plan for a week. Recipes for the starred items are in Chapter 9 Recipes.

Note the use of leftovers including dinner leftovers for lunch, Roasted Vegetables for the Beet Salad, Stir-Fry Vegetables to make Vegetable Frittata, and Chili for the Mexican Tostada Salad.

Emily Iker Meal Plan

Emily Iker has secondary lymphedema of the leg and typically eats meals similar to these.

Breakfast:

- Kefir, small cup

- Orange, half

- Either eggs (hard boiled or fried), cereal, or a small fruit or vegetable pancake made with whole grain mix, egg, milk, and grated vegetable (squash, carrot, etc.) or fruit.

- Coffee

Morning Snack:

- Slice of cucumber, apple, mango

Lunch:

- Salad with salmon or chicken

Afternoon Snack:

- Mixed nuts: about 6 nuts

Dinner:

- Small portion of fish or chicken; grass-fed beef steak every two weeks

- Potatoes (small boiled) or brown rice

- Broccoli or other vegetables

- Tea: jasmine/green tea, chamomile, or rose hip

Linda-Anne Kahn Meal Plan

Linda-Anne Kahn has lipedema and typically eats a mix of foods similar to those shown in Table 8-2 on page 135.

Linda-Anne plans on:

- Snacks: nuts (hazel nuts, cashews, pecans, walnuts), hummus, raw vegetables, chocolate with 70% cacao, coconut water, or goat kefir

- Soups: about four nights a week, vegetable, lentil, bean, or cauliflower

- Red wine: occasionally, 5 ounces or less

- Water: at least 10 ounces each day

Table 8-1: Recommended Meal Plan

Meal	Day 1	Day 2	Day 3	Day 4	Day 5	Day 6	Day 7
Breakfast	Oatmeal, Banana (half), Kefir	Corn Tortilla with nut butter, Banana (half), Kefir	Oatmeal, Banana (half), Kefir	Corn Tortilla with nut butter, Banana (half), Kefir	Vegetable Frittata, Orange, Kefir	Oatmeal, Banana (half), Kefir	Vegetable Frittata, Orange, Kefir
Lunch	Salad Niçoise*, Orange	Ratatouille*, Orange	Beet Salad*, Orange	Kale with Sweet Potato*, Orange	Veggie Stir-Fry*, Banana (half)	Salmon Salad, Vegetable Soup, Orange	Mexican Tostada Salad*, Banana (half)
Dinner	Ratatouille* with beans	Roasted Vegetables*	Kale with Sweet Potato*	Veggie Stir-Fry* with beans	Vegetable Soup*, Bean Salad*	Chili*, Napa Cabbage Slaw*	Pasta-Less Primavera*

- Sauerkraut: 1 tablespoon about 5 days a week

- Avocado: about 5 times a week

- Brown rice and tofu: occasionally at restaurants with no other choices

Planning Tips

General Guidelines

Keep these ideas in mind when making meal plans:

- Variety: strive for many different vegetables and fruits including those that are in season. Try new varieties.

- Carbohydrate: have some carbohydrate at each meal and more than one type of carbohydrate (beans, fruit, starchy vegetables, whole grains) each day.

- Fruits: at least two servings each day, including citrus and banana.

- Omega-3 foods: fatty fish at least twice a week (if you eat fish)

- Kefir: 4 ounces of kefir morning and evening can help improve gut dysbiosis.

- Animal products: limited animal products to 6-8 servings week. Servings are 3-4 ounces of cooked meat, 2 eggs, 8 ounces of milk, or 1.5 ounces of cheese.

Food quantities should be reasonable for your size. For most people this means at least a half-cup of beans plus a half-cup of whole grains (such as oats), a cup of starchy vegetables, or one cup of fruit each day.

Adequate protein is not a concern, meals with a mixture of beans and other plant-based carbohydrate will typically provide enough protein.

Meal Planning

Meal planning for this eating plan may be different, especially if you currently plan around the protein at the center of the plate.

Table 8-2: Linda-Anne Kahn Meal Plan

Meal	Day 1	Day 2	Day 3	Day 4	Day 5	Day 6	Day 7
Breakfast	Omelet with 2 eggs, tomatoes, cilantro	Smoothie*	Eggs fried in butter (2)	Smoothie*	Goat kefir with strawberries	Smoothie*	Goat kefir with blueberries
Lunch	Vegetable Soup*, Salad with butternut squash	Hard-boiled eggs (2), Rice crackers	Salad, tomatoes, sprouts, cucumbers	Lentil Salad, Brazil nuts (6), Coconut water	Orange, apple, and nuts	Salad	Quinoa salad with vegetables
Dinner	Salmon salad, tomatoes, cucumbers, sprouts, avocadoes	Salmon, zucchini, beets, arugula, sauerkraut	Quinoa black bean patties (2), broccoli	Lentil soup and kale salad, avocado	Vegetable Stir Fry* with broccoli, maitake and shitake mushrooms, quinoa	Kale salad, Curried vegetables	Vegetable Soup*, Yam salad

Try these ideas:

- Focus on a favorite flavor, spice, or ethnic food as the theme for a meal. Recipes can be prepared with a variety of different flavors.

- Give pride of place on the plate to vegetables, especially seasonal treats.

- Include three or more bright colors (other than white, brown, and beige) at each meal.

- See "Transition Aids" on page 142 for tips on replacing bread, pasta, and meat.

- Consider alternatives to favorite foods in "Eat This/Not That" on page 207.

Carb Counting

If you find it difficult to figure out food types and quantities for meals, try planning based on carbohydrates (see "Carbohydrate Counting" on page 226):

- Decide how many grams of net carbohydrates you would like each day, based on your desired calorie intake (check with your health care provider or a dietitian). For example 200 grams per day.

- Set a carbohydrate target for each meal and snacks that adds up to your daily total. For example, 45 grams for breakfast, 60 grams for lunch, 75 grams for dinner, and 20 grams for snacks.

- Plan the carbohydrate part of each meal to meet your target. For example, breakfast with 45 grams of carbohydrate could include half a grapefruit (11 grams), half a banana (12 grams), and a cup of oatmeal (24 grams).

- Fill out the rest of your meal with no- or low-carbohydrate foods. For example, coffee, tea, or almond milk (unsweetened).

Counting carbohydrates is simpler than counting calories because many foods—such as non-starchy vegetables, tofu, eggs, nuts, or meats—contain little or no carbohydrate. For example, a salad or stir-fry with a variety of low carb vegetables and canned garbanzo beans can be evaluated based on the carbohydrate in the beans only; a one half cup serving of beans is about 15 grams of net carb (total carb minus fiber).

Budgeting based on carbohydrates gives you flexibility to make trade-offs. For example, if you replace oatmeal with scrambled tofu and vegetables—which have no carb—you can use the 24 grams of carbs you saved at another meal on the same day.

Soup-to-Nuts

Starting a meal with soup, salad, or both is a good way to blunt hunger and fill up on low carb vegetables. Soups are easy to make (see "Soups" on page 156) and a good way to use leftovers or extra vegetables. Most soups freeze well, soups frozen in serving or meal-sized containers will be more convenient and thaw faster.

Nuts (raw or dry roasted, no sugar or salt) make a nice way to end a meal and provide a healthy alternative to grain- or dairy-based sweet desserts.

Make Ahead

Making foods in advance or in larger quantities (planned-overs not left-overs) may mean that you do not have to cook as often. Extras from dinner make great lunches or salad toppings. Freeze anything that will not be used within 5-7 days.

Here are some suggestions:

- Bean salads* are easy to make, keep well, and can be used as a side dish, entrée or salad topping.

- Caramelized onions* and sautéed peppers* add flavor and color to salads (arugula, goat cheese, onions, walnuts), soups, stir-fry, wraps, etc.

- Oatmeal can be refrigerated or frozen in meal-sized portions and heated in the microwave.

- Salad Dressings* with healthy fats, low sodium, and no additives are easy to make and keep well.

- Soups, especially Chili* which can be used in multiple dishes..

- Vegetable frittata* is a baked egg casserole that can be part of any meal and is simple to make. Save time by fixing extra vegetables for a meal and using some vegetables for a frittata that bakes while you are eating..

- Vegetable salad* or chopped salad makes a good side dish or salad topping.

Menu Suggestions

Menu items for different eating occasions. Recipes are provided for items marked with an asterisk (see Chapter 9).

Breakfast

Fruit:

- Citrus: grapefruit or orange
- Banana (half)
- Berries

Grains or beans:

- Oatmeal
- Granola
- Whole grain cereal (gluten-free)
- Corn tortilla toasted or fried (dry) with nut butter or goat cheese
- Bean Burrito* or Bean Salad*

Other:

- Smoothie*
- Vegetable Frittata* or other egg dishes
- Kefir
- Coffee or tea

Lunch

Here are some lunch ideas, in addition our dinner suggestions and leftovers:

- Soups
- Vegetables, raw or blanched

- Salads with vegetables, beans, salmon, tuna, non-gluten grains, etc.

- Wraps with corn tortillas or lettuce leaves filled with vegetables, beans, tuna, tofu, tempeh, etc.

- Bean Spread* or hummus with corn tortilla, oat crackers, or flatbread

- Pickles, sauerkraut, and other fermented vegetables

- Fruit: orange, apple, berries

Dinner

Entrees:

- Veggie Stir-Fry* with beans, brown rice, or other whole grain

- Ratatouille*

- Roasted Vegetables*

- Kale with Sweet Potatoes*

- Pasta-Less Primavera*

- Vegetable Frittata*

- Beet Salad*

- Mexican Tostada*

- Salad Niçoise*

Side Dishes:

- Bean Salad*

- Blanched Vegetables*

- Napa Cabbage Slaw*

- Southwestern Potato Salad*

Soups:

- Chili*

- Pea Soup*

- Vegetable Soup*

Desserts

- Berries, try kefir as a topping.
- Fruit
- Hot Fruit Dessert*
- Almond Cake*
- Coconut Ice Cream, in small quantities
- Dark chocolate
- Nuts

Light Snacks

Try lighter snacks when you want something but are not that hungry:

- Vegetables: including carrots, celery, snap peas, snow peas, Jicama, kohlrabi, daikon, radishes, baby turnips, etc.
- Blanched Vegetables*
- Raw cabbage or lettuce.
- Pumpkin seeds (try with chili powder), sunflower seeds, etc.
- Water (with citrus for flavor)
- Unsweetened tea
- Coconut water
- Crystalized ginger (small amount) or ginger tea
- Tiny candies: savor one flavorful piece

Substantial Snacks

Snacks containing carb or protein for times when you are hungry:

- Nuts: 1 ounce or 1/4 cup of raw unsalted nuts. Premeasure into serving size packets for help tracking quantities; also mind the limit on Brazil nuts (see "Selenium" on page 98).

- Trail mix: find a version without candy or crackers, or make your own.
- Granola: look for oat-based granola without too much sweetener or rice.
- Fruit: small citrus fruit, stone fruits, apple, berries, etc.
- Dried fruit or berries, in small quantities
- Kefir or plain yogurt
- Bean Spread* or hummus with oat- or rice-crackers
- Corn tortilla
- Soybeans or edamame
- Orange juice
- Bean Salad*

Potluck or Family Gathering

These recipes work well for larger groups and parties.

- Brussels Sprouts with Lemon*
- Winter Squash Medley*
- White Beans and Fennel*
- Oriental Green Beans*
- Bean Salads*
- Broccoli Salad*
- Crudité Platter*
- Marinated Mushrooms*
- Napa Cabbage Slaw*
- Southwestern Potato Salad*

Transition Aids

Here are some suggestions for moving away from bread, pasta, and meat.

Bread Alternatives

Bread that contains less gluten can help with the transition away from wheat-based foods. For example, Ezekiel brand multigrain breads (sold refrigerated or frozen).

Not eating bread means replacing sandwiches with wraps made using leaves, tortillas, or other wrappers. Corn tortillas are a versatile alternative that can be used soft (steamed or heated) or crispy (toasted or fried). Tortillas are made from coarsely ground corn (masa). Corn tortillas are generally not gluten free because flour is used to keep them from sticking together.

Oat based crackers or flatbread are other versatile alternatives. Brown-rice crackers can be tasty but check the carbs and sodium content.

Gluten free cornbread mix is one of the few gluten-free foods that is not full of rice or tapioca starch. Look for a mix where you have to add sugar and use half the sugar specified on the package, optionally add canned or frozen corn or peppers.

Pasta Alternatives

Several foods can replace pasta:

- Beans are good, especially meaty lima beans (gigantes), and they are easy to add to pasta sauce for a one-dish meal.

- Spaghetti squash cooked by baking or steaming breaks into sweet strands that look like spaghetti.

- Black bean pasta is one of the few gluten-free pasta alternatives that does not contain rice or tapioca starch.

- Polenta made with corn or quinoa is available in ready-to-eat packages.

Meat Substitutes

Vegetarian meat alternatives can be helpful during the transition to eating smaller amounts of animal products. Meat substitutes are highly processed foods that may be high in sodium or contain food additives.

Most meat-replacements are soy or gluten based. The more desirable soy products are made from tempeh or tofu. Other more highly processed forms of soy include soy protein isolate, texturized soy protein, or texturized vegetable protein.

Gluten based products may be labeled seitan or wheat-meat. Gluten looks and chews more like meat than other meat substitutes. However, gluten is off-limits for anyone with gluten sensitivity.

Plain tempeh is one of the healthier and more economical options. Tempeh has with a nice chewy texture but needs sauce for more flavor and visual appeal. Use grated or finely chopped tempeh in place of ground meat in sauces.

Savory or meaty flavor (umami) comes from an amino acid in meats. The same amino acid is found in mushrooms, tomatoes, aged cheeses (such as Parmigiano-Reggiano), and fermented foods like fish sauce or soy sauce.

Use these foods to provide or enhance umami taste:

- Big Portobello mushrooms as a burger alternative with a little tamari soy sauce.

- Mushrooms and tamari soy sauce topping for other burger alternatives.

- Savory dishes with cremini mushrooms, tomatoes, and aged cheeses.

Chapter 9

Recipes

Use these recipes to get started with our recommended eating plan. Feel free to adapt them for your tastes and your available ingredients.

About these recipes:

- Tastes: recipes are mild with are options for strong and varied tastes provided in "Sauces and Flavorings" on page 185. Try the basic recipe and then adjust the flavors to suit.

- Cooking oils: recipes call for olive oil but coconut oil can be used in equal amounts for cooking, if the taste is acceptable. You may want different types of olive oil for cooking and salad dressings.

- Vegetables and fruits: these recipes can be used with many different types of vegetables and fruits. Specific preparation instructions are in Chapter 10.

- Red onions are used in these recipes because they are colorful and tasty. White or yellow onions can be used instead.

- Salt and sodium: most of these recipes are good without adding any salt and we provide an extensive list of low-sodium seasoning options.

Main Dishes

Quick and easy one-dish meals, Quantities are for two people, with left-overs, unless otherwise noted.

Vegetable Stir Fry

This core recipe allows many variations with different combinations of vegetables, sauce or flavor elements, and (optional) starch or protein. We have it frequently but it is never the same.

Any of the sauces or flavors (see "Sauces and Flavorings" on page 185) can be used with stir-fry. Mostly we do not add anything or add ginger and a little tamari soy sauce.

Variations with additional starch or protein:

- Add canned or pre-cooked beans for a one-dish meal: garbanzo beans, black beans, small white beans, etc.

- Serve over brown rice, quinoa, or oatmeal.

- Mix in pre-cooked or ready-to-eat brown rice, quinoa, or other grain.

- Add 1-2 eggs per person during the last part of cooking, along with sauce or flavor, and cook until eggs are firm. Either crack the eggs into the pan and stir to mix, or scramble eggs before adding.

- Add chopped tofu, tempeh, or meat substitute during the last part of cooking.

You can use almost any assortment of vegetables or just one vegetable in addition to the onion, garlic and carrot. We use 4-6 cups of vegetables but quantities are flexible (as long as they fit your pan).

Notes on vegetable choices:

- Red onions work well with all tastes and provides more color.

- Eggplant: long thin varieties of eggplant (Chinese, Japanese, or Thai) work well and cook more quickly than wide Italian eggplant. You may have to add oil repeatedly when cooking eggplant, especially the Italian variety.

- Starchy vegetables such as potatoes, beets and other root vegetables, or winter squash must be in small pieces to cook completely in a stir-fry.

The secret to cooking many types of vegetables together is to start the longer cooking vegetables first, and then progressively add vegetables with shorter cooking times, so they are not overcooked. You can prepare everything before you start cooking or prep ingredients in cooking order, and add them when they are ready.

General guidelines for timing:

- First: onion, carrot, leek, garlic
- Second hard/starchy vegetables: cauliflower, Brussels sprouts, broccoli, root vegetables
- Third soft vegetables: eggplant, summer squash, peppers, beans, asparagus
- Fourth fast cooking vegetables: snap peas, snow peas, bok choy, spinach, other leafy vegetables, mushrooms, bean sprouts, cabbage

Ingredients (one example):

- Olive oil
- Onion 1 medium red onion and/or 1 medium leek, chopped
- Garlic: 2-3 cloves, minced
- Carrot: 1 medium, chopped
- Cauliflower: about 1 cup chopped
- Zucchini: 1 medium, chopped
- Yellow squash: 1 medium chopped
- Snap peas: 1 cup trimmed and chopped
- Red cabbage: 1 cup chopped.

Directions:

- Heat 1-2 tbsp. of oil in the wok or frying pan until hot.
- Add onion or leek, garlic, and carrots.
- Fry over medium heat, stirring occasionally.
- When onions look softened, add the cauliflower.
- When cauliflower starts to look translucent, add the zucchini and squash

- Stir frequently, adjust the heat, and add oil if needed.

- After about 5 minutes, add the snap peas and cabbage.

- Cook about another 5 minutes, until the peas are bright green and the cabbage wilts.

- Add any sauce or flavor elements.

Ratatouille

Ratatouille is a versatile eggplant stew that is good hot or cold and can be an appetizer, entrée, or side dish. Ingredients and quantities are flexible.

Variations:

- Serve over brown rice, quinoa, or oatmeal as an entrée.

- Add beans or cooked potatoes for a one-dish meal.

- Add grated or cubed cheese when serving.

Ingredients:

- Olive oil

- Onion: red onion and/or leek, chopped

- Garlic: 3 or more cloves, minced

- Carrots: 1 or 2 cut into thick coins or chunks

- Celery: 1 stalk chopped

- Eggplant: 2 medium or one large Italian eggplant, diced with skin on

- Zucchini: 1 diced

- Yellow squash: 1 diced

- Cauliflower (optional): 1 cup chopped.

- Mushrooms (optional): 1 cup or more chopped.

- Tomatoes: either fresh 3-4 cups chopped; no salt added canned 28 ounces (one 28 ounce or two 14-ounce cans) petite cut, chopped, or ground tomatoes or a mix of tomatoes and tomato sauce or puree.

- Fresh or dried herbs, such as bay leaf, to taste.

Directions:

- Heat 2 tbsp. of olive oil in a large pot until hot.

- Add garlic, carrots, onion, and cauliflower and cook until onions wilt.

- Add eggplant and cook on medium heat stirring frequently and adding more olive oil as needed (eggplant absorbs oil as it cooks).

- When the eggplant starts to look cooked, (color changes from white to gray) add the yellow squash, zucchini and mushrooms.

- When the vegetables are just about cooked (not too well done) add the tomatoes and simmer for 15 minutes or more.

- Adjust the spicing before serving. May need a little sugar if too acid.

Roasted Vegetables

Roasted vegetables make a great meal on a cold night. Left overs are good cold or can be added to other dishes such as Beet Salad.

Roasted garlic is soft, mild, and tasty. Consider roasting extra garlic for use as a flavoring in other dishes or salad dressings.

Quantities are flexible and one baking sheet holds about 7-8 cups of chopped vegetables. We usually make three sheets worth, one for each time range. If you make more than your oven will hold in one batch, plan on additional time.

Parchment paper for cooking is sold in rolls and makes cleanup from roasting vegetables much easier. Look for it in the baking supplies section of the grocery store.

Our recipe calls for crushed garlic in olive oil to coat the vegetables. If you do not have a garlic press, use minced garlic or garlic flavored oil. Fix the oil before preparing the vegetables so the oil can absorb the flavors.

There are different opinions on the best temperature for roasting vegetables, with some recipes going as high as 450 or 500°F. Higher temperatures shorten the cooking time and brown vegetables more but can easily burn them. Lower temperatures are more forgiving and less likely to form cancer-promoting chemical compounds. We recommend 375° but you can increase to 425° if you are in a hurry.

Similar to stir-fry, the secret to roasting vegetables is to start the longer-cooking vegetables first and add the vegetables with shorter cooking times later, so everything finishes at the same time. Cooking times are flexible; if something looks done early, take it out of the oven.

Plan on at least an hour of baking time for harder vegetables. Softer vegetables need less cooking time and can be prepared while longer cooking vegetables are baking.

Longer cooking time (60 minutes):

- Potatoes: red, yellow, purple

- Beets

- Onions: red onions cut into quarters or thick disks and held together with a toothpick

- Carrots

- Garlic cloves, peeled

- Leeks: use small leeks, cut off bottom (roots), outside leaves, and most of green top.

Medium cooking time (45 minutes):

- Sweet potato

- Sweet peppers: red, orange or green cut into strips

- Winter squash (Kabocha, Acorn, other) cut into slices and peeled.

- Brussels sprouts trimmed and cut in half

Faster cooking (30 minutes):

- Cauliflower sliced into bite size chunks

- Broccoli

- Summer squash

- Asparagus

- Turnips

- Eggplant

- Mushrooms

- Tomatoes, cut and squeeze out juice

Ingredients (in addition to the roasting vegetables):

- Olive oil

- Garlic

- Salt (optional)

- Rosemary, other herbs or spices, or balsamic vinegar (optional)

Instructions:

- Preheat the oven to 375°F.

- Prepare baking sheets or pans. If not using non-stick pans, line with parchment paper or lightly coat bottom with oil.

- Pour 2 tbsp. of olive oil in a large container (7-8 quarts) with a lid.

- Crush 1-2 cloves of garlic in a garlic press, or mince, and add to the oil.

- Add a little salt to the oil (optional)

- Add rosemary, other herbs or spices, or balsamic vinegar to the oil (optional)

- Fill container with cut vegetables, close, and shake to coat vegetables with oil mixture.

- Empty onto baking sheet and spread out into a single layer.

- Bake as directed until vegetables are tender.

Kale with Sweet Potato

Quick and easy to prepare and very versatile. Served hot as a main dish or room temperature as a salad. Be careful not to cook the greens too long, so they stay bright.

Variations include:

- Use other potatoes (red, yellow, purple, etc.), winter squash, or a mix.

- Replace kale with chard or other greens.

- Add chopped tempeh or tofu near the end of the cooking time.

Ingredients:

- Olive oil

- Onion: 1 large red onion, sliced thin

- Garlic: 3-4 cloves, minced

- Carrots: 2 carrots, chopped

- Sweet potato: 1 large or 2 small, chopped

- Kale: 1 bunch prepped and chopped (see "Kale" on page 195)

- Tamari or soy sauce (optional)

- Salt and pepper (optional)

Instructions:

- Heat oil in a large frying pan with a lid.

- Sauté onions, carrots, and garlic until the onion begins to brown

- Add sweet potato and simmer covered, stirring occasionally and adding oil if needed.

- When sweet potatoes are starting to get soft, add the kale, mix and simmer for a few minutes. The kale should wilt but remain green and slightly chewy.

Pasta-Less Primavera

Pasta primavera adapted into a one-dish meal with beans, or as a sauce over polenta, spaghetti squash, or black bean pasta. The combination of tomatoes, mushrooms, and grated cheese give this dish a savory umami taste. Serve with chard or other greens.

Ready-to-eat polenta rolls are available in several flavors including varieties made from quinoa and corn. Any other type of polenta would also work. Check sodium content on packaged foods or mixes.

Variations on this dish include:

- Vegetables: almost any combination of vegetables can be used including asparagus, eggplant, zucchini or other summer squash, cauliflower, etc.

- Tomatoes: fresh or canned tomatoes. Fire roasted tomatoes or other chopped tomatoes work well (drain some of the liquid), stewed tomatoes can be drained and mixed with tomato puree or paste for thicker sauce.

- Starch: mix in beans (gigantes, garbanzo beans, any other canned or cooked beans) or serve over polenta, spaghetti squash (see "Spaghetti Squash" on page 179), or black bean pasta (prepared according to the instructions on the package).

Ingredients:

- Olive oil

- Onion: 1 large red onion, sliced thin

- Garlic: 3-4 cloves, minced

- Carrots: 2 carrots, chopped

- Vegetables: 3-4 cups, bite size pieces

- Mushrooms: 6 or more medium brown mushrooms, sliced

- Starch: 14 ounce canned beans, drained, 2 cups cooked beans, or Polenta 16 ounce roll

- Tomatoes: 14 ounce can fire roasted, chopped, or stewed tomatoes or 2-3 cups of fresh tomatoes, chopped and drained

- Basil fresh or dried (optional)

- Salt and pepper (optional) or red pepper flakes

- Sugar (optional)

- Grated cheese (optional)

Instructions for heating polenta roll:

- Pre-heat oven to 300°F

- Slice polenta roll into 8-10 disks and put on a baking sheet.

- Heat while preparing sauce, turning once.

Instructions for sauce:

- Heat 1-2 tbsp. of oil in a large frying pan.

- Sauté onions, carrots, and garlic until the onion softens

- Add vegetables and cook, stirring occasionally, add oil if needed (eggplant absorbs oil)

- When vegetables have softened, add mushrooms

- When mushroom start to look cooked, add the tomatoes, beans (if using beans), and basil.

- Simmer until flavors are blended, and fresh tomatoes have cooked down

- Adjust seasoning if needed, add a little sugar if too bland or harsh.

- Serve over polenta (2-3 disks per serving) or spaghetti squash

- Top with grated cheese.

Vegetable Frittata

Vegetable Frittata is a baked egg dish that is easy to make, can take on many different flavors, works well for any meal, and is good hot or at room temperature. Frittata is an easy way to make eggs for a large group.

There are many options for different tastes based on:

- Vegetable filling: stir-fry mixture of onion, carrot, broccoli, cauliflower, red cabbage, mushrooms, etc.

- Flavor element mixed with the eggs: hot sauce, mustard, sun-dried tomatoes, mild chilies, grated cheese, etc.

- Topping (optional): grated cheddar, parmesan, dry jack or other cheese.

- Sauce (at serving time, optional): Caramelized Onions*, Sautéed Peppers*, tomato sauce, salsa, hot sauce, etc.

Vegetable filling is lightly cooked Vegetable Stir-Fry*. One timesaving tip is to make a large stir-fry for dinner, use some of the vegetables to make frittata, and bake the frittata while you are eating. Smaller pieces of vegetables work better for frittata. Remove the vegetables for the frittata when they are just barely cooked and before adding sauce to the stir-fry.

Any favorite vegetables can be used in the filling but filling should be dry or the frittata will be mushy. If the filling includes vegetables that release water during cooking–such as tomatoes, mushrooms, or peppers–drain the vegetables before adding to the frittata.

The number of eggs need will vary depending on the size of the eggs and the quantity of vegetables. Egg mixture should cover the vegetables completely. A thicker frittata provides more servings and takes longer to bake.

Ingredients:

- Olive oil

- Eggs: 6-10 as discussed above.

- Filling: 3-4 cups of stir-fried vegetable mixture as discussed above.

- Flavor element (optional): as discussed above.

- Topping (optional): cheddar, parmesan, dry jack, etc.

- Sauce (optional): as discussed above

Instructions:

- Pre-heat the oven to 350 degrees.

- Wipe the inside of a 9" square baking dish with olive oil or other anti-stick product.

- Stir-fry the vegetable filling.

- Break the eggs into a bowl and beat the eggs.

- Add the optional flavor element to the eggs and mix.

- Put the vegetable filling into the baking dish, should be about half-full (3/4" deep).

- Pour in the egg mixture and stir gently to blend. Beat and mix in more eggs, if needed to over the vegetables.

- Sprinkle cheese on top (optional).

- Bake until eggs are firm in the center, about 30 minutes (depending on thickness). Brown briefly under the broiler, if needed.

- Serve with (optional) sauce.

Soups

These hearty soups can be a main course or part of a meal.

Pointers:

- Watch the salt content if you use pre-made broth (which is not necessary); select low-sodium broth and/or dilute the broth with water.

- Most soups freeze well. Soups in serving or meal-sized containers will be more convenient and thaw faster.

Vegetable Soup

Another recipe that allows many variations in terms of ingredients and flavors. Soup is a great use for extra vegetables or leftovers.

Add ingredients based on cooking time: long cooking starchy ingredients, medium cooking time non-starchy vegetables, and then fast cooking greens. The timing is flexible, and undercooking is best for most ingredients.

Fresh or dried kidney beans are the exception and should boil for at least 10 minutes. Frozen beans may only be blanched (check the label); if so, they need more cooking. Canned beans are fully cooked and can be added near the end of the cooking time.

Brown rice takes about 45 minutes to cook. For a quick soup, use pre-cooked rice and add the rice near the end of the cooking time.

Long cooking starchy ingredients include:

- Potatoes: 1-4 cups of bite size pieces.

- Beans: 1-4 cups of fresh, frozen, or dried and pre-soaked.

- Brown rice: about 1 cup of raw rice.

- Winter squash: 1-4 cups of cubes.

- Beets, turnips, rutabagas, and parsnips: 1-4 cups.

- Medium cooking time vegetables include:
- Cauliflower
- Broccoli
- Zucchini or yellow squash
- Mushrooms

Fast cooking greens include Bok choy, cabbage, escarole, spinach, Swiss chard, Snap peas, snow peas, or English peas, etc.

Ingredients:

- Olive oil
- Low Sodium vegetable or chicken broth: quart or 48 ounces
- Onion and/or leeks: 1 medium red onion and/or 1 leek, chopped
- Garlic: 2-4 cloves, minced
- Carrots: 2 carrots, cut into thick coins.
- Celery: 1 stalk, chopped
- Bay leaf (optional)
- Other herbs and spices (optional)
- Starchy vegetables (optional): see above
- Medium cooking time vegetables (optional): see above
- Greens (optional): see above

Instructions:

- Heat 1-2 tbsp. of olive oil in a large pot.
- Add onion or leek, garlic, carrots, celery and sauté until onion is soft.
- Add broth, bay leaf, and long-cooking starchy vegetables; bring to a boil.
- Turn down and simmer until vegetables are almost tender.
- Add medium cooking time vegetables, cooked beans, and cooked rice.

- Simmer until vegetables are lightly cooked.

- Add other herbs and spices.

- Add greens and simmer. Thin light greens such as spinach cook instantly, thicker greens like kale need more cooking time.

- Adjust seasoning, if necessary.

Variations:

- Use stewed or chopped tomatoes and tomato sauce or juice in place of broth.

- Use more beans and less broth for a bean soup.

- Add beets and cabbage for borscht.

- Blend part or all of the soup for a creamier base.

Chili

Chili make a hearty main dish or soup. Chili can also be used for the bean mixture in a Mexican Tostada Salad* or Bean Burrito*.

Flavor can range from mild, almost sweet, to fiery. If you are cooking for people with varied tastes, make the chili mild and serve it with hot sauce, salsa, onions, or peppers for those who want more heat.

Adjust the balance between vegetables and beans based on the menu. Use more vegetables than beans for a one-dish meal, or more beans when served with salad or other vegetable dishes. Use many types of colorful vegetables including those with stronger tastes. For examples, broccoli, Brussels sprouts, and cauliflower.

Choice of beans or mix of beans can also vary. Use only red kidney beans for a traditional chili, black beans for black bean chili, or multiple types of beans including garbanzo and lima beans (gigantes). Canned beans are fast and easy; drain off extra liquid before adding beans, or rinse if the beans are high salt.

Cooking fresh or dried beans thoroughly is important for minimizing gas and other digestive issues. Dried beans should be pre-soaked overnight, and the soaking water discarded. Do not taste fresh or dried kidney beans until they have boiled for 10 minutes.

For fresh beans, or dried beans that have been soaked, either boil the beans for 10 minutes before adding them to the chili or change the cooking sequence and extend the cooking time. Add uncooked beans before the vegetables and boil the beans for at least 10 minutes before tasting them. Add the vegetables after the beans have boiled so the vegetables will not be overcooked.

Fresh, canned or frozen corn, including varieties with red and green peppers, adds color (and other types of amino acids). Add corn near the end of the cooking time because it cooks quickly.

Prepared chili powder is an easy way to get a basic chili taste, look for a good quality powder that does not contain salt or is low in salt. For more flavor depth and heat, add hot peppers or chilies that are fresh, dried, or canned.

Ingredients:

- Olive oil

- Onion: red onion chopped

- Garlic: 3-4 cloves, minced

- Carrot: 1 medium, chopped

- Celery: 1 rib diced

- Vegetables: 3-4 cups, chopped

- Beans: 28 ounces (2 14 ounce cans) drained canned beans, 3-4 cups of presoaked dried beans, or 3-4 cups of fresh beans. Boil fresh or dried kidney beans for 10 minutes before tasting the beans or adding them.

- Tomatoes: 28 ounces no-salt canned tomatoes petite cut, chopped, or ground tomatoes or a mix of tomatoes and tomato sauce or puree

- Corn (optional): fresh, canned, or frozen corn kernels

- Spices: chili powder

- Peppers (optional): red pepper flakes, chilies, or hot peppers

- Avocado (optional) for garnish, peeled and sliced

Instructions:

- Heat 1-2 tbsp. of oil in a large pot
- Add onion, garlic, carrot and celery and sauté until onion is wilted
- Add chopped vegetables and cook for about 10 minutes (vegetables should not be fully cooked)
- Add beans, tomatoes, and corn and heat until boiling
- With canned beans, this only need to boil briefly; fresh or dried beans should be boiled until fully cooked
- Turn heat down to simmer
- Add chili powder and peppers to taste. Start conservatively, you can add more spice later.
- Simmer at least 15 minutes and adjust the spice.
- Serve garnished with avocado slices.

Pea Soup

This recipe includes soaking the dried peas overnight. If you are not able to soak overnight, you can skip that step and simmer them longer until they cook completely.

Ingredients:

- Split peas: 16 ounces or more
- Low Sodium vegetable or chicken broth: quart or 48 oz
- Carrots: 2, cut into thick coins.
- Potatoes: 3 medium red or equivalent in smaller or larger potatoes, cut into bite size pieces.
- Onion and/or leeks: chopped to taste
- Garlic: chopped to taste

Empty peas into large pot and add broth. Add additional water to cover if needed. Bring to a boil, turn off, cool, and refrigerate overnight. Add more broth or water to cover peas, if needed (peas will absorb water and expand).

Add remaining ingredients to soup. Add more water to cover if needed. Bring to a boil and then simmer for 30 minutes or more until the potatoes are cooked and the peas are soft.

Variations:

- Add fresh or frozen green peas or snap peas just before serving.

- Add corn or tomatoes to soup.

- Add fresh or dried mint.

Salads

Beet Salad

Arugula has a slightly bitter taste that pairs well with something sweet like beets. In this recipe, beets, crunchy walnuts, and smooth goat cheese provide a variety of tastes and textures.

Good beets are the secret to this salad. You can roast them yourself (see "Roasted Vegetables" on page 149) or you may be able to buy precooked beets or beet salad.

If beets are not available, substitute other roasted vegetables or Caramelized Onions*.

Ingredients:

- Arugula

- Beets (roasted beets, precooked beets, or beet salad)

- Goat cheese

- Walnuts: whole or pieces

- Oil: walnut oil or extra virgin olive oil

- Vinegar: sherry or balsamic vinegar

Directions:

- Toast walnuts (see "Toasted Nuts" on page 182)

- Fill salad bowls with arugula

- Top with beets

- Dot with goat cheese
- Sprinkle on walnuts
- Dress with oil and vinegar

Salad Niçoise

Salad Niçoise is a classic composed salad with many variations.

Ingredients:

- Greens: arugula or romaine work well
- Fish: canned tuna, tuna salad, seared tuna (available pre-cooked), anchovies, or salmon
- Starch: small boiled potatoes or large lima beans (gigantes)
- Olives (optional): traditionally ripe Niçoise olives cured in brine and packed in olive oil but any ripe or green olives can be used.
- Egg (optional): hard-boiled egg, quartered or sliced
- Vegetables: blanched French beans, asparagus, or other vegetables
- Dressing: oil and vinegar or vinaigrette

Directions:

- Fill salad bowls with greens
- Arrange fish, starch, and vegetables
- Top with eggs, olives, and dressing

Mexican Tostada Salad

Mexican style salad with a base of beans and a crispy corn tortilla. Can be made with the "Mexican Bean Mixture" on page 182, leftover "Chili" on page 158, or refried beans.

Tostada ingredients:

- Lettuce: chopped romaine lettuce
- Corn tortilla: one per salad

- Beans: Mexican Bean Mixture, Chili, or other beans.

- Taco sauce

- Guacamole

- Tomatoes (optional): sliced tomatoes

- Salsa fresca or pico de gallo (optional): mixture of fresh chopped tomatoes, onions, cilantro, hot green peppers, salt, and lime juice.

- Salsa (optional)

Directions for tostada:

- Heat corn tortilla in toaster oven, oven, or dry frying pan until crisp.

- Place tortilla in the bottom of each salad bowl.

- Cover with warm Mexican Bean Mixture.

- Fill bowl with lettuce

- Top with tomato slices, guacamole, salsa fresca, and taco sauce

- Serve with salsa

Bean Salads

Bean salads can be a side dish, a salad topping, snack, or even part of break-fast. Salads can be one type of bean (garbanzo bean salad, kidney bean salad), mixtures of beans (three bean salad), or beans and corn (black beans and corn salad). You can buy mixtures of beans (salad beans) or create your own combinations.

For example:

- Garbanzo bean salad with olive oil, balsamic vinegar, chopped green onion, whole grain mustard, salt, and pepper.

- Three-bean salad with kidney beans, garbanzo beans, string beans, olive oil, wine vinegar, parsley, salt, and pepper.

- Black-bean salad with black beans, canned corn, chopped sweet pepper, lime juice, cumin, and Mexican hot sauce.

Use fully cooked beans, such as canned beans. Frozen beans may only be blanched (check the label) if so they should be boiled briefly for salad. Soak dried beans overnight, discard the water, add fresh water and boil until fully cooked. Fresh or dried kidney beans must be boiled for 10 minutes before using or even tasting.

Ingredients:

- Olive oil

- Vinegar

- Beans: any mixture of cooked or canned beans

- Vegetable accents (optional): green onion, blanched carrot, green bean, snap peas, etc.

- Spices and flavors

Instructions:

- Add oil, vinegar, spices and flavors to a container with a tight-fitting lid.

- Mix together, taste, and adjust flavor.

- Add beans and vegetable accents.

- Close lid and shake to coat beans with dressing.

- Refrigerate until ready to use.

Broccoli Salad

Basic vegetable salad that can be prepared in advance. Use with different color and flavor accents for variety.

Example color and flavor accents:

- Toasted walnuts or slivered almonds (see "Toasted Nuts" on page 182)

- Caramelized Onions* and Sautéed Peppers*

- Orange and yellow for fall, with grated carrot and sweet orange or yellow peppers

- Red peppers for Christmas, use chopped fresh sweet peppers, chopped pimento or marinated sweet peppers

Ingredients:

- Broccoli: one or more bunches of broccoli, chopped and blanched (see "Blanched Vegetables" on page 183).

- Color and flavor accent: as discussed above.

- Salad dressing: any oil and vinegar based dressing (see "Salad Dressings" on page 184)

Instructions:

- Combine all ingredients and mix well. Chill before serving.

Crudité Platter

Great for an appetizer, starter, or potluck. See the instructions for "Blanched Vegetables" on page 183 and the instructions for preparing vegetables in Chapter 10.

- Asparagus: blanched

- Broccoli, all varieties, blanched

- Cauliflower: raw or blanched

- Celery

- Cucumber sticks

- Daikon or other radishes

- Endive leaves (good for dips)

- Fennel slices

- Green beans: blanched

- Jicama sticks

- Kohlrabi sticks

- Mushrooms: plan or marinated (recipe below)

- Peppers: all colors of sweet peppers or mild peppers

- Snap peas, snow peas, edible pod peas, blanched

- Zucchini or summer squash sticks

Variations:

• Dips: see "Dips or Spreads" on page 185

• Mexican or Southwestern: drizzle with lime or lemon juice and dust with smoked paprika, chili powder, or cayenne (depending on your taste for spice).

Marinated Mushrooms

Quick appetizer or salad ingredient. Marinate mushrooms for 1-3 hours before serving. The marinade discolors the mushrooms over time.

Variations:

• Marinate in other vinaigrette-type dressings for different tastes. See "Salad Dressings" on page 184.

• Mix in other Blanched Vegetables*

Ingredients:

• Mushrooms: 1 quart of cleaned white or button mushrooms in bite-sized pieces.

• Olive oil: 3 tbsp.

• Vinegar: 1 tbsp. light vinegar: apple cider, Champagne, rice wine, white wine, etc. or juice of 1 Meyer lemon, if available.

• Mustard: 1 tsp. sharp mustard such as Chinese, Dijon, English, etc.

• Garlic: 1 small clove crushed in a garlic press or minced fine, or roast garlic.

• Pepper: white pepper if available.

• Salt (optional)

• Sugar (optional)

Instructions:

- Mix the marinade in a quart container with a tightly fitting lid.

- Taste the marinade on a piece of mushroom and adjust seasonings. May need a little sugar or water if too strong.

- Add the mushrooms, seal the lid, and shake to coat mushrooms.

- Refrigerate and shake periodically.

Napa Cabbage Slaw

Tasty alternative to traditional coleslaw with a lighter texture. Any coleslaw dressing or vinaigrette can be used. Makes about 7 cups.

Ingredients:

- Napa cabbage: 1 head, chopped

- Red cabbage: 1/4 head, chopped

- Carrot: 1 carrot, grated or finely chopped

- Yogurt: about 1/2 cup plain yogurt

- Lemon juice: juice of 1-2 fresh lemons (Meyer lemon, if available); can substitute any light vinegar.

- Pepper (optional): white pepper if available.

- Salt (optional)

- Sugar (optional)

Instructions:

- Mix the yogurt and lemon juice in the bottom of a large bowl.

- Taste and adjust seasoning, dressing should be pleasantly tart.

- Add the vegetables and mix well.

- Transfer to a container with a tightly fitting lid and refrigerate.

Southwestern Potato Salad

Southwestern style salad with a variety of tastes and colors. Potatoes and carrots can be cooked in advance, but avocado and other ingredients should be added just before serving.

Ingredients:

- Sweet potatoes: 4 medium or 7 cups diced
- White potatoes: 4-6 to provide 3 cups diced
- Carrots: 2 large or 1 cup coins
- Canned corn: Southwestern Style (black beans and peppers), Mexican Style (peppers), or regular, drained; or blanched frozen corn kernels or fresh corn. Add canned black beans (rinsed and drained), if not using Southwestern corn.
- Avocado: 1 or 2 peeled and chopped
- Olive oil
- Limes: 2 limes, juiced
- Cilantro (optional): chopped leaves ¼ to ½ cup
- Chili powder (optional)
- Salt (optional)
- Pepper or hot sauce (optional)

Directions:

- Boil sweet potatoes until just tender, rinse and cool
- Boil white potatoes and carrots until just tender, rinse and cool
- Combine all ingredients in large bowl and mix.
- Adjust seasoning to taste.

Vegetable Salad

Vegetable salad or chopped salad makes a good salad, side dish, salad topping, or snack. This salad can be made in advance and will keep for a few days but the (optional) garnish should be added just before serving.

Ingredients:

- Vegetables: mix of raw or blanched diced vegetables such as carrots, celery, broccoli, green onion, zucchini, cauliflower, cucumber, sweet peppers, mushrooms, tomatoes, etc.

- Dressing: oil and vinegar, homemade Salad Dressing*, or other dressing.

- Garnish (optional): avocado slices, other diced fruit, seeds, or nuts.

Instructions:

- Mix vegetables and dressing in a container with a tight fitting lid.

- Chill to allow flavors to meld.

- Add (optional) garnish just before serving.

Side Dishes

White Beans and Fennel

This hearty dish works well for a potluck or as a side dish. Orange and fennel are a classic flavor combination that contrast nicely with the sweet beans.

If sectioning oranges is too much trouble, remove the seeds and chop the flesh.

Ingredients:

- Olive oil

- Onion: 1 large or 2 medium red onions, diced

- Garlic: 3-4 cloves, minced

- Carrot: 1 or 2, diced

- Fennel: 1 large bulb, chopped

- White beans: 2-3 14 ounce cans of small white beans, drained

- Orange: 2-3 juice oranges, sectioned and chopped (see page 199)

- Salt (optional)

- Pepper or red pepper flakes (optional)

Instructions:

- Heat 1-2 tbsp. of olive oil in a large frying pan.

- Sauté the onion, garlic, and carrot until the onion is soft.

- Add the chopped fennel and cook briefly. Fennel should remain crunchy.

- Add the beans and spices.

- Simmer for 15-20 minutes and adjust the spices.

- Mix in the orange segments and remove from heat.

Oriental Green Beans

This dish can be made using one or more types of green beans such as Italian or Romano beans, long beans, string beans, snap peas, snow peas, etc. Chop the green beans into bite-sized pieces. If you are using multiple types of beans, keep the varieties segregated.

Add the longer cooking Italian or Romano beans first, followed by string beans. Snap peas and snow peas cook quickly and should be added last.

Ingredients:

- Olive oil

- Garlic: 2-4 cloves, minced

- Carrot (optional): 1 carrot diced

- Green beans: several cups of one or more varieties

- Tamari soy sauce (optional)

- Ginger (optional): minced

- Sesame seeds (optional)

- Sesame oil (optional)

Instructions:

- Heat oil in a wok or frying pan with a lid.

- Brown garlic and carrot and lightly while preparing the green beans.

- Add longer cooking beans and ginger, cover and steam a few minutes.

- When long cooking beans start to become tender, add other beans.

- When beans are lightly cooked, toss with tamari sauce, sesame seeds, and sesame oil and remove from heat.

Winter Squash Medley

This recipe makes a tasty squash medley that can be a main course or side dish. Dried berries and nuts make a festive addition for holiday gatherings. The mix of winter squash and other vegetables is very flexible.

Ingredients:

- Olive oil

- Onion and/or leeks: 2 red onions or 1 onion and 1 leek, chopped

- Garlic: 3-6 cloves, minced

- Carrots: 2 carrots, chopped

- Winter squash: 4-8 cups of any combination of Delicata, Kabocha, butternut, etc. cut into bite sized pieces. See page 198 for prep instructions.

- Dried Berries (optional): currants, raisins, or cranberries (reduced sugar)

- Nuts (optional): chopped nuts such as pecans or walnuts

- Other vegetables (optional) as desired, such as mushrooms, sweet pepper, red cabbage, snap peas, summer squash, etc. Canned garbanzo beans, or small white beans are also good.

- Seasoning (optional): sherry, Marsala, or other sweet wine, tomato sauce or tomato puree, cinnamon, curry or Moroccan spices

Instructions:

- Heat 1-2 tbsp. of oil in a large frying pan (with a lid).

- Add onion, leek, and garlic and sauté over medium heat until wilted.

- Add carrots, squash, along with the berries or nuts, if you are using them.
- Cover and simmer, stirring frequently. Adjust the heat and add a little oil or liquid if needed.
- When squash starts to get soft, add seasoning and other vegetables and mix.
- If other vegetables include greens, you may want to cover the pan to steam them.
- Can be reheated on the stovetop or in the oven. Add sherry or sweet wine if it seems too dry.

Sweet Potato Casserole

Sorry, no marshmallows but easy to make and tasty. Can use any combination of sweet potato, yam, and winter squash.

Ingredients:

- Sweet potato, yam or winter squash (any combination): 6-8 cups of bite size pieces
- Carrots: 2-3 carrots in bite size pieces
- Dried fruit: 1/2-1 cup of chopped dried apricot, cherries, cranberries, etc.
- Orange juice: 1-2 cups
- Cinnamon (optional): to taste

Baking instructions:

- Heat oven to 375°F.
- Mix ingredients in a large bowl
- Transfer to a shallow baking dish
- Bake until tender, stirring occasionally, about 30 minutes

Wok Steamed Greens

Steaming is a quick way to prepare greens as a side dish or for a wilted salad. Use for broccoli (all varieties), chard, collard greens, kale, mustard greens, pea shoots (pea plants), spinach, etc.

Greens should be washed and slightly damp (shake off excess water) for steaming. If they are too dry, add a little water. If they are too damp, you may have to drain them after they are cooked.

Ingredients:

- Olive oil

- Garlic: 2-4 cloves, minced

- Greens: one bunch of greens, chopped (see prep instructions in Chapter 10).

Instructions:

- Pour 1-2 tbsp. of oil into the wok

- Add the garlic and let marinate while you prepare the greens.

- If you have stems, add them to the wok now.

- Heat the oil, garlic and (optional) stems on medium heat.

- When the garlic begins to brown, add the greens, cover tightly, and reduce heat.

- Check and stir every couple of minutes, greens wilt and cook down quickly.

- Remove from heat and take off the lid when greens look barely cooked. Taste a stem or piece if you are not sure.

Optional variations:

- Pine nuts or slivered almonds: brown along with the garlic.

- Fresh ginger: chop finely and add along with the greens.

- Tamari soy sauce: splash a little at the end.

- Balsamic vinegar or balsamic glaze, add a small amount at the table.

Brussels Sprouts with Lemon

This recipe makes a large dish suitable for potlucks or family gatherings. Good hot or at room temperature.

Three options for the lemon element, each with a different taste:

- Preserved lemon is a North African ingredient made of small whole lemons pickled in brine for an intense lemon flavor. You can find these at specialty stores or online.

- Meyer lemons have a sweet/tart taste and a great aroma and can be used raw (wash in hot water first). These are seasonal and may be hard to find.

- Regular lemon that are pre-cooked for a sweeter taste: wash in hot water, slice 1/4" thick, remove seeds, cover with water and boil for 2 minutes, and drain.

Ingredients:

- Olive oil

- Onion: 1 large red onion, diced

- Garlic: 4-6 cloves, minced

- Carrot: 1 large carrot, diced

- Brussels sprouts: 2 pounds of Brussels sprouts. Cut small spouts in half and larger sprouts in quarters so pieces are small and will cook quickly.

- Slivered almonds: 1/2 cup slivered almonds

- Lemon: one medium lemon (to taste), either preserved, Meyer, or pre-cooked.

- Dried apricots: 4 dried almonds, chopped

- Salt and pepper (optional)

Instructions:

- Cover dried apricots with hot water and let soak to soften.

- Toast slivered almonds in a frying pan (no oil needed), toaster oven or oven until slightly browned.

- Heat olive oil in wok or large frying pan.

- Add onion, garlic, and carrot; brown onion while you prepare the Brussels sprouts.

- Sauté the Brussels sprouts over medium-high heat until just tender and slightly browned. Add more oil if needed.

- Cut lemon in half, move seeds and chop.

- Add the lemon, almonds, and apricots the Brussels sprouts.

- Taste and adjust seasonings. Add a little brine from the preserved lemon if it needs salt or more lemon flavor.

Desserts

Almond Cake

Gluten free cake with a great almond/coconut taste that is good plain or with fruit or berry topping.

Full recipe makes 18 servings (9x13 inch pan); half makes 9 servings (8x8 inch pan).

Ingredients:

- Sugar: 1/2 cup

- Almond meal/flour: 1 1/2 cups or about 6 oz

- Coconut flour: 1/2 cup or about 1 oz

- Baking powder: 2 tsp

- EITHER butter: 3/4 cup salted butter (1 1/2 sticks) OR coconut oil: 3/4 cup and salt: 1/4 tsp salt

- Eggs: 4

- Almond extract: 1 tsp (increase for more almond taste)

- Milk: 1/2 cup, can use unsweetened almond milk

- Vanilla extract: 1 tsp

- Coconut (optional): shredded coconut can be mixed in or used as topping
- Almonds (optional): slivered almonds for topping

Instructions:

- Preheat oven to 350 °F.
- Prepare glass baking dish by lining with foil or wiping with butter
- Blend all dry ingredients together in a large bowl
- Melt butter or coconut oil in microwave for 30 seconds or in hot water
- Mix into dry ingredients.
- Beat eggs with milk and extracts
- Mix into dry ingredients and blend until creamy
- Spread batter in pan
- Top with (optional) almonds or coconut
- Bake for 30 minutes or more, until center is firm
- Serve with fruit or berry topping

Hot Fruit Dessert

Hot fruit makes a tasty treat for dessert or a topping for other dishes. This is overkill for ripe luscious fruit but works well for fruit that is uninteresting and needs a little more sugar. Try adding cinnamon after heating.

Works with: apples, pears, peaches and other stone fruit, etc.

- Slice the fruit thinly and remove any bruised areas

Microwave:

- Spread the slices in a single layer on a plate.
- Cover and cook until hot, about 30-60 seconds (depending on microwave)

Stove top:

- Spread slices in a single layer on the bottom of a dry frying pan.
- Heat pan for a few minutes on medium heat, until fruit is hot, turn fruit once.

Other Recipes

Some of these foods are used in other recipes or as flavor accents.

Smoothie

Smoothie makes an easy breakfast or other meal.

Ingredients:

- Protein powder: 2 scoops (tablespoon) of complete dairy free protein powder
- Goji berries: 1 tablespoon
- Maqui berry powder: 1 tablespoon
- Greens: about 1 cup of kale or spinach leaves
- Cucumber: 2 small Persian cucumbers or 1/4 of a long English cucumber
- Bee pollen: 1 tablespoon
- Berries: handful of fresh or frozen raspberries, strawberries, blueberries
- Salmon oil: 1 tablespoon
- Almonds: 6 nuts
- Almond milk or coconut milk beverage: 1/2 cup
- Flax seeds/chia seeds/hemp seeds: 1 tablespoon
- Water: 1/2 cup cold water

Directions:

- Put ingredients into a heavy-duty blender or food processor
- Blend until smooth
- Drink immediately

Bean Burritos

These little bean burritos can be used for breakfast, lunch, or as a side dish.

Variations: for a breakfast burrito, use a smaller amount of beans and add a scrambled egg.

Ingredients:

- "Mexican Bean Mixture" on page 182
- Corn tortillas: one per burrito
- Lettuce (optional): shredded lettuce or cabbage
- Chopped Tomatoes or Salsa Fresca (optional)
- Salsa (optional)

Microwave instructions:

- Put tortilla on a microwave-safe plate and top with 2-4 tbsp. of bean mixture.
- Cover and heat for 30-60 seconds (depending on microwave).
- Top with optional ingredients and roll into burrito shape.

Stove top instructions:

- Heat bean mixture in a saucepan
- Sprinkle drops of water on a tortilla and heat in a dry frying pan until soft.
- Place 2-4 tbsp. of bean mixture in the center.
- Top with optional ingredients and roll into burrito shape.

Cornbread

Gluten free cornbread mix is one of the only gluten-free products not loaded with rice or tapioca starch. However, these mixes can be high in sugar. If the mix calls for adding sugar, try using one-half or three-quarters of the recommended amount.

Ingredients:

* Gluten free cornbread mix: 1 package

* Corn: 1 14-15 ounce can of Mexican Style corn with peppers or plain canned corn, drained; or 2 cups cooked fresh or frozen corn kernels.

Instructions:

* Prepare cornbread per package instructions (may require egg, butter, sugar, etc.), using less than the recommended amount of sugar.

* Mix in drained canned corn just before pouring batter in the baking dish..

* Bake per package instructions (may require additional baking time).

Spaghetti Squash

Spaghetti squash can cooked by baking or steaming to soften the flesh. Once cooked, the flesh can be scraped out to form spaghetti like strands. The strands have a mild, pleasant flavor.

Ingredients:

* Spaghetti squash: one squash cut in half-lengthwise with seeds removed.

Baking instructions:

* Heat oven to 375°F.

* Place squash cut side down in a large, shallow baking dish, and add a little water to the dish. Optionally cover with aluminum foil.

* Bake for 30-45 minutes (depending on the size of the squash) and check if the flesh separates easily into spaghetti-like strands. If not, bake for another 10 minutes and check again.

- Allow squash to cool enough to handle, and scrape the flesh out of the shell.

- Serve, or mix into sauce, immediately.

Steaming instructions:

- Put about 1/2" of water and a steamer rack in the bottom of a large pot.

- Add the spaghetti squash cut side down.

- Boil for 30-45 minutes (depending on the size of the squash) and check if the flesh separates easily into spaghetti-like strands. If not, boil for another 10 minutes and check again.

- Allow squash to cool enough to handle, and scrape the flesh out of the shell.

- Serve, or mix into sauce, immediately.

Caramelized Onions and Sautéed Peppers

Caramelized onions and sautéed peppers provide a sweet and crunchy flavor accent for use hot on burgers, or cold on salads, sandwiches, or wraps. Cooked onions keep well; make these in advance or make extra for leftovers. Quantities are flexible and you can make only onions or peppers.

Ingredients:

- Olive oil

- Onions: 1 large or 2 small red onions, thinly sliced. Use a mandolin or a food processor to slice larger quantities.

- Garlic (optional): 2-3 cloves, minced

- Carrots (optional): 1 carrot, diced

- Sweet pepper: 1 sweet red pepper, cleaned and sliced

Directions:

- Heat heavy frying pan (with a lid) on low

- Add onions, garlic, carrot, and sweet pepper

- Cover and stir occasionally until onions are soft and sweet. Add olive oil or water, if too dry.

Bean Spread

Bean spread similar to hummus that works well as a dip, in a wrap, or sandwich. Walnuts give white beans a slightly bluish tint. Can be made with any type of beans, or mixture of beans. Try all small white beans (navy beans) or a mix of navy beans and garbanzo beans for a more interesting texture.

Makes about 4 cups.

Ingredients:

- Beans: 4 cups of cooked beans or 2 14 ounce cans of beans, drained.

- Green onion: 1 green onion (mostly the green part), chopped

- Garlic: 1-2 cloves, minced or roasted garlic puree

- Lemon juice: juice of 2 lemons or about 1/3 cup

- Walnuts: 2/3 cup walnut pieces

- Dill (optional): fresh dill or 1/2 tsp dried dill

- Salt or tamari soy sauce (optional)

- Hot sauce, pepper, or other flavors (optional)

Instructions:

- Put walnuts in food processor and pulse to chop coarsely

- Add remaining ingredients (except salt and hot sauce) and puree until almost smooth.

- Taste and adjust seasonings.

Mexican Bean Mixture

Use this Mexican bean mixture for Mexican Tostada Salad, Bean Burritos, as a side dish or added to salads. Keeps well and can be made in larger quantities.

Ingredients:

- Olive oil
- Onion: 1 small red onion or half a large onion, minced
- Garlic: 1-2 cloves, minced
- Beans: 1 can (14 oz) black beans or pinto beans, drained, or 2 cups of dried beans that have been soaked and cooked
- Chili powder (optional)
- Cumin (optional)
- Salt (optional)
- Pepper or hot sauce (optional)

Instructions:

- Heat 1 tbsp. olive oil in a frying pan.
- Sauté onion and garlic until tender
- Add the beans and spices, mix together and mash some beans
- Simmer at least 10 minutes, stirring occasionally
- Adjust the spices and add salt and pepper or hot sauce to your taste

Toasted Nuts

Toasting helps bring out the flavor in nuts. Toast just before using or serving.

- Spread a single layer of nuts in a small frying pan and heat on low.
- Check for doneness and shake or stir periodically. Usually about 10 minutes.

For large quantities, toast in a 300°F oven or toaster oven on low.

Cranberry Orange Relish

This fresh relish is very tasty and versatile but not too sweet. We have served it with turkey, duck breast, and cornbread.

Ingredients:

- Cranberries (fresh or frozen and thawed): 12 ounce bag
- Oranges: 2-3 juice oranges
- Sugar

Directions:

- Dump cranberries in cold water and pick out spoiled berries and stems.
- Drain cranberries and transfer to a saucepan with a lid.
- Wash two oranges in hot water and scrape orange zest onto the berries.
- Juice the oranges; add juice and some orange pulp to the berries.
- If needed, juice additional oranges, until the juice covers the berries.
- Cover pan and heat on medium heat until mixture boils and berries pop.
- Turn heat low, stir occasionally and mash any un-popped berries.
- When berries are popped (about 10 minutes), turn off and cool.
- Taste and add just enough sugar to be pleasantly tart, about 2 tablespoons.

Blanched Vegetables

Blanching brings out the sweetness in vegetables (making them more acceptable to kids) while keeping their bright colors and crunchy texture. This is a fast, easy way to prepare vegetables for use as snacks, in salads, or with dips.

Most vegetables only need a few seconds in boiling water. Remove vegetables before they are fully ready because they can continue to cook. Use an ice-water bath to chill vegetables if you are doing a large quantity.

Good for: asparagus, broccoli, cauliflower, carrots, green beans, kale, snap peas, snow peas, sweet peppers, etc. Timing is easier to manage if you do each type of vegetable separately.

Directions:

- Boil a pot of lightly salted water large enough to hold the vegetables.

- Prepare a colander to receive the blanched vegetables and optionally a bowl of ice water.

- Prepare vegetables per the instructions (see Chapter 10).

- When the water is boiling, add the vegetables.

- After about 30 seconds, remove a sample, rinse in cold water and taste.

- As soon as the vegetables are almost done, transfer the vegetables to the colander.

- Rinse with cold water or transfer to the ice-water bath.

- Drain vegetables.

Salad Dressings

Homemade salad dressings are easy and better for you in terms of healthy fats, less sodium and sugar, and no additives. Oil and vinegar is the easiest.

Vinaigrette type dressings are easily mixed in a shaker bottle and keep well. Try different combinations of these parts:

- Oil: walnut oil, olive oil, avocado oil, etc. Coconut oil is solid at room temperature and not useful for salad dressing.

- Acid: different flavors of vinegar, lemon, lime, or orange juice, etc.

- Flavorings: garlic, ginger, soy, mustards, tomato paste, fresh herbs, etc. and spices peppers, curry, paprika, etc.

The classic ratio is three parts oil to one part acid or vinegar. You may prefer more vinegar, depending on the ingredients you are using.

Olive oil based dressings may solidify in the refrigerator. This is normal and the dressing will turn liquid again when it warms up to room temperature.

Dips or Spreads

Mix plain yogurt with different flavor elements to make dips or spreads. Try different brands of Greek yogurt, regular yogurt, or a combination to get the right consistency for dip.

For example:

- Onion dip with chopped Caramelized Onions* and tamari soy sauce.

- Spinach dip with finely chopped spinach cooked with leek and garlic.

- Ranch dip with fresh dill, horseradish, and white pepper.

- Mustard dip with Dijon or whole grain mustard.

- Curry dip with curry powder or a mix of curry spices such as coriander, cumin, fenugreek, ginger, turmeric, and chili pepper.

Sauces and Flavorings

Spices can be health promoting and recommended foods can be as spicy as you like. Use these suggestions to quickly and easily add favorite flavors and new tastes, without excessive sodium.

General suggestions:

- Taste before adding anything. The natural flavors in our recipes may not require flavoring or salt, depending on your tastes.

- Use sauces sparingly and add just before serving, especially sauces containing sweeteners and salt. A tablespoon or two can flavor a whole dish; add a little water, sherry, or low-sodium broth if you need more sauce or the taste is too strong.

- Start cautiously, adding more flavor is easier than correcting for too much.

- Adding sauce at the table lets everyone pick their own favorite flavors. Leftovers prepared without sauce can have different flavors.

- Check the ingredient list for allergens. Look for alternative versions, if you need them, such as vegetarian oyster sauce or Worcestershire sauce.

- Instant sauces or soup mixes are often high sodium and contain food additives, check the labels.

Try these flavor elements for a wide range of different tastes:

- Bottled sauces are available in a wide variety of flavors including variations of barbeque, Chinese, Indian, Japanese, Mexican, Thai, etc.

- Broth, including low-sodium broth, adds a little flavor and salt taste. You can use broth by itself or to dilute other sauces.

- Cheeses can provide savory umami taste (aged Parmigiano-Reggiano), salty accents (cheddar or feta), or cool smoothness (goat cheese).

- Citrus juices, rind or flesh provide a variety of tastes and smells ranging from tart to sweet, depending on the variety of citrus and the cooking time. Try juice or flesh from lemon, Meyer lemon, lime, orange, or other varieties.

- Coconut milk provides a rich flavor in sauces that are sweet or spicy. Try coconut milk, fresh lime juice, and curry powder for a Thai taste.

- Dried fruits such as apricots, cranberries (reduced sugar), currants, etc. keep well and add interesting tastes. Chop apricots and other larger fruit; pre-soak dried fruits in hot water if they are hard.

- Fruit provides interesting flavors or contrasting tastes. For example, tart apples with braised red cabbage, or sweet fruits with a spicy curry.

- Garlic is good fresh (in small amounts) or roasted (see Roasted Vegetables) which has a very mild flavor. Prepared garlic is available in several forms including roasted garlic puree.

- Ginger is very tasty and health promoting. If fresh ginger is not available, you can use finely chopped crystalized ginger or ginger powder.

- Hot sauce or pepper sauce comes in many different varieties, each with a taste associated with certain cuisines. For robust flavors that are not overwhelming, try small amounts of hot sauce that is not vinegar based.

- Mushrooms add savory taste (umami) and texture. Try cooking with fresh dark mushrooms (portobello, cremini or button) or small amounts of dried mushrooms (porcini, shiitake, other) that have been soaked in water, rinsed, and chopped.

- Mustards add taste to many dishes including salad dressings, dips, marinades, egg dishes, etc. Try whole grain, Chinese, Dijon, English, Russian, and other varieties with different flavors.

- Nuts add taste and texture to salads and hot dishes.

- Oils provide different tastes for salad dressings and marinades, try walnut oil (plain or toasted), extra-virgin olive oil, flavored oils infused with herbs, garlic, lemon, orange, truffles, etc. Add toasted sesame oil just before serving for an oriental taste and aroma.

- Peppers and chilies that are fresh, dried, or canned provide a range of flavors, especially in small quantities. Keep strong chilies, such as smoked chipotle peppers, in the freezer and shave off a little as needed.

- Salt taste from wheat-free soy sauce (tamari) or Braggs Amino (available in a spray bottle) provides more savory flavor depth (umami) than salt.

- Soups or entrées from heat and serve packages (check the sodium content), take-out, or leftovers make tasty toppings for stir-fry or steamed vegetables. For example, Indian lentil dahl or Thai coconut soup.

- Spices and herbs for your favorite flavors, here are some basics: bay leaves, black pepper, chili powder, cinnamon, and curry powder. Buy in small quantities so they stay fresh.

- Sugar or maple syrup (in small amounts) can be useful for adjusting and improving flavors. For example, if a tomato-based sauce seems acid or harsh; one teaspoon of sugar can balance the taste and give the flavor more depth.

- Tomato can add flavor depth and savory taste (umami) in small amounts without making tomato the dominant taste. Try small amounts of tomato paste (available in tubes), tomato sauce (8 ounce cans), sun-dried tomatoes, tomato chutney, catsup, etc.

- Vinegars of different types or infused with flavors provide different tastes for salad dressings, marinades, and savory dishes. Balsamic glaze is an interesting condiment for greens or berries.

- Wines including Marsala (or other sweet wines), red wine, or sherry add interesting taste and flavor depth. Avoid cooking wines with added salt.

- Yogurt or kefir can be used to make sauces (such as curry), as condiments, or for flavor interest in many dishes. If a dish is too spicy for your tastes, try balancing the heat with yogurt.

Chapter 10

Preparing Vegetables and Fruits

Whole foods do not come with instructions and we encourage you to try many different varieties. Here are pointers on how to prepare fresh vegetables and fruits.

Vegetables

Asparagus

Asparagus spears should be stiff and crisp when raw but may have a tough and woody area near the base. Asparagus can be eaten raw but is usually blanched or cooked which makes it sweeter.

- Cut across the bundle of asparagus to trim the ends of all the stems.

- Put the cut ends in a bowl of cold water until you are ready.

- Rinse the asparagus in cold water.

- Discard any spears that are shriveled, limp, or decayed.

- Snap off and discard the tough base end. If the end does not snap move up closer to the tip.

Leave spears whole if you are going to blanch them or cook them separately.

Cut into smaller pieces for stir-fry or soup:

- Spread spears out in one layer with bases roughly aligned.

- Slice on a diagonal to make pieces that are about 1/2 thick.

Beets, Turnips, Rutabagas

Root vegetables are sometimes sold with their bottom root and tops (stems and green leaves) attached. Tender greens can be used in soups or other dishes.

- Cut off the small bottom root where it connects to the bulb.

- Trim off the top where it connects to the bulb.

- Wash off any remaining dirt and trim off any small roots.

Beets or turnips that will be eaten raw should be scrubbed or peeled. Peeling is optional for vegetables that will be cooked. Turnips and rutabagas from retail stores may be coated with edible food-grade wax that can be moved by peeling. Be careful with raw beets because the juice can stain clothing or cutting boards..

Bell Pepper/Sweet Pepper

- Turn the pepper upside down and slice down through the center.

- Separate the halves and tear or cut out the green top and central seed cluster.

- Remove any fleshy ribs.

- Rinse inside and out to remove loose seeds.

Bok Choy

Bok choy vary widely in size, the whole plant can be eaten.

- Trim ends and wash, checking for dirt in the leaves.

- Baby bok choy (under 3"): cut in half or quarters lengthwise.

- Larger bok choy: cut in half lengthwise and chop into 1/2" slices.

Broccoli

Broccoli grows as a thick stalk with florets at the top. Broccoli may be small and tender (sometimes labelled baby broccoli or broccolini) or pre-trimmed (broccoli florets with very little stem) in which case you can use it all.

Thick stalks can be tough and bitter, so you may only want to use the top part of the stem. Trim off the base and cut a piece of stem to taste, if you are not sure.

- Remove leaves and their stems.

- Rinse broccoli and trim off any discolored florets.

- For cooking by itself: slice vertically into spears.

- For mixed dishes: cut florets into bite size pieces and stems into 1/2" slices.

Brussels Sprouts

Brussels sprouts look like little cabbages but they grow on all sides of a large stem.

- If sprouts are on the stem, cut each one off where it attaches to the stem. Discard the stem.

- Trim the base of each stem and cut off any damaged areas.

- Pull off loose or wilted outer leaves.

- For stir-fry: cut large sprouts in half or quarters vertically so that small sprouts and pieces of large sprouts are roughly the same size.

Cabbage or Napa Cabbage

- Rinse and remove any damaged outer leaves

- Stand on stem and cut into quarters vertically

- Slice out the stem.

- Chop by slicing finely, starting from the base, and cross-cutting.

Carrots

Carrots should be washed but peeling is optional. Green tops from carrots are sometimes used in soups.

- Trim off the top and bottom.
- Cut out any bad areas.
- If the carrots are thick and you need small pieces, slice lenghtwise.
- For roasting: cut 1-3" chunks.
- For salads or frittata: cut into small pieces.
- For soups: cut into 1/2" thick coins.
- For stir-fry: chop coarsely.

Cauliflower

Cauliflower grows in a tight head with multiple florets surrounded by leaves.

- Rinse the cauliflower, if necessary.
- Trim any discoloration off the florets.
- Turn the cauliflower upside down,
- Cut off the leaves at the stem, remove and discard.
- Separate florets by cutting them off the central stem.
- Chop florets into bite sized pieces and trim the stems.

Chard

Chard is a big leafy vegetable with a broad stem. The stems are edible but may need more cooking time than the leaves.

- Trim the ends of the stems and put in cold water until ready to use.
- Rinse the leaves; tear out and discard any damaged areas.
- Stack the leaves and cut the stems off.
- Chop the stems into 1/4" slices and set aside.

- Roll the leaves into a giant cigar shape.
- Slice crosswise every 1/4".
- Chop coarsely in the other direction.

Eggplant

There are many varieties of eggplant with different shapes. All can be cooked with the skin on.

- Rinse eggplant, trim off the top, any leaves, and the bottom.
- Indian eggplant (egg size and shape): dice.
- Italian eggplant (fat): cut into 1/2" slices vertically, then dice.
- Oriental eggplant (long): slide in halves or quarters lengthwise, then dice.

Fennel

Fennel is a white bulb topped by green stalks with feathery green leaves. The stalks look like celery and the leaves look like dill but they smell like anise.

- Trim off the bottom and the green stems on top.
- Rinse the fennel bulb.
- Remove any damaged spot or the outer layer, if it does not look good.
- Slice vertically into four pieces.
- Finely slice each piece horizontally.

Garlic

A head of garlic contains clusters of cloves encased in papery white skin. Both the size of the head and the size of the individual cloves can vary considerably. Outer cloves are larger than inner cloves, and some cloves may be too small to peel and use.

The quantity of garlic depends upon your tastes and the dish. Start with one clove for two servings.

- Peel off the outer skin of the head and break out the number of good-sized cloves you need.
- Trim off the top and bottom of each clove.
- Remove the papery skin around the clove; it may help to score it vertically.
- Slice the cloves vertically into a couple of pieces.
- Lay the slices flat and mince by cutting in both directions.

If you are using a garlic press:

- Slice the cloves horizontally into a couple of pieces.
- Stack these slices in the garlic press and squeeze the handles.

Ginger Root

Look for ginger roots that are firm and not dry looking (shriveled). The amount of ginger you need will depend on your tastes, the size of the dish you are making, and how strong the ginger tastes.

- Trim off one end of the root.
- Cutting towards the cut end, remove 1/2 to 3/4" of skin on all sides of the root.
- Turn root sideways, and slice as thinly as you can, cutting parallel to your original cut. This may be difficult because you are cutting across the fibers.
- Lay the slices flat and mince by cutting in both directions.

Jicama

Jicama has light brown skin and white flesh and is usually eaten raw.

- Rinse the jicama.
- Cut off the top and bottom.
- Remove the skin by pulling, peeling or cutting.
- Cut the flesh into sticks for snacks or salads.

Kale

Baby kale leaves can be eaten whole. Large kale leaves (all varieties) have a tough center stem that should be removed before eating. Kale can be eaten raw, blanched, or cooked. Raw kale is sometimes massaged to soften it up for salad.

- Trim the ends of the kale and let stand in cold water until ready.
- Rinse the kale and remove any bad leaves or areas.

There are several ways to remove the stem:

- Cut on either side of the stem.
- Pull the stem through a plastic stem stripper device.
- Grasp the stem with one hand and pull with the other, using your hand as the stripper device.

After stems have been removed:

- Chop the kale by rolling into a big cigar shape, slicing every 1/4", and then chopping coarsely in the other direction.

Kohlrabi

Kohlrabi can have a tough skin with a crisp interior that is usually eaten raw:

- Remove any stems and leaves from the bulb.
- Position the stem on the left side of the bulb.

- Slice down vertically about 1/2" from the left and right sides to remove the top and bottom.

- Stand the kohlrabi on one cut end.

- Cut downward around the outside to remove the rest of the peel. Turn it over and work from both ends.

- For snacks: cut into slices or sticks.

Leeks

Leeks look like giant green onions but are cooked before eating. Green parts at the top can be tough and may be discarded.

- Trim the base to remove the roots or a small amount of the end.

- If the outer layer is limp or damaged, strip it off.

- Wash the leek, checking the spaces at the top that may contain dirt.

- For cooking separately: leave whole or cut to fit pan.

- For roasting: cut into 2" sections.

- For other uses: slice cross-wise into 1/4" disks, discard top parts if dirty.

Mushrooms

Prepare mushrooms just before cooking or serving.

- Cut off the bottom 1/4" of the stems and any damaged areas.

- Rinse and brush off any visible dirt.

- Cut into quarters, slices, or leave whole.

Onions or Shallots

Remove the dry outer layers of onions before chopping or cooking:

- Position the onion with the root on the left and the top on the right.

- Slice down vertically about 1/2" from the left and right ends to remove the bottom and top,

- Cut vertically through the outer layer only.

- Peel off the outer layer.
- Remove additional layers if there is damage or spoilage.

Cut depending on desired result:

- Quarters for roasting: cut down vertically from top to bottom. Insert wooden toothpicks before slicing to hold quarters together.
- Rounds: position with top to your left and slice vertically, slice thin for serving raw, about 1/2" thick for roasting.
- Strings: slice in half vertically, place cut side down, top to the left, and slice finely.
- Diced: slice in half vertically, place cut side down, top towards you, make slices that stop about 1/4" short of the bottom, turn top to the left and slice finely.

Potatoes, Sweet Potatoes, Yams

Potatoes of all varieties can be cooked and eaten skin and all, without being peeled.

- Wash potatoes
- Cut out any bad spots or remaining dirt

Radishes or Daikon

- Trim off tops, bottom roots, any side roots (look like hairs).
- Scrub clean.

Spinach

Baby spinach is often pre-washed and the stems can be left on. Check for and remove any spoiled leaves and re-wash if you find spoilage.

Full size spinach is often sold with roots attached, must be washed carefully, and should have the stems removed.

- Cut off the root end of the stems and let stand in cold water until ready.
- Tear off and discard the stems.

- Vigorously agitate the leaves in a bowl of cold water.

- Scoop out the leaves, leaving the water in the bowl.

- Check the bottom of the bowl for sand or dirt, if you find any refill the bowl with clean water and repeat the process until all the sand is gone.

- For cooking: roll leaves into a big cigar shape; slice every 1/4", then chop coarsely in the other direction.

Summer Squash

Summer squash include zucchini, yellow squash, etc. and can be eaten raw or cooked. Very large zucchini have seeds the center that can be scooped out before cooking.

- Rinse and trim off both ends:

- Dice: cut in quarters (or smaller) lengthwise, then chop.

- Coin: cut 1/4" thick crosswise.

Winter Squash

Winter or hard squash come in many varieties, including cooking or sugar pumpkins, and are cooked before eating. Squash may be coated with edible wax, depending on where you buy them. These varieties can be cooked and eaten with the skin on (if not waxed): delicata, kabocha, but these have tougher skins: acorn, butternut, Hubbard, pumpkin, and spaghetti squash.

General instructions:

- Cut in half vertically through the stem.

- Scoop out seeds and tendrils with a grapefruit spoon.

- Baking: just leave in halves.

- Roast veg: cut into 1/2" slices and then cut off skin (if necessary).

- Dice: slice (and optionally skin) as for roast veg, then cut into bite sizes.

Fruits

Avocado

Avocados have a tough outer skin and one large pit in the lower part of the fruit. A ripe avocado will give a little bit when squeezed. Avocados are usually eaten raw or added to cooked dishes just before serving.

- Cut the avocado in half, cutting down from the top (smallest end) and cutting around the pit with a small knife.

- Separate the two halves by twisting them and pulling them apart.

- Remove the pit by cutting into it with the knife and twisting it free.

- Use a soupspoon, about the size of the large end, to scoop out the inside of each half.

- Trim off any dark bad spots.

- Slice lengthwise into wedges or chunks.

Grapefruit

To cut a grapefruit in half before serving:

- Position the scar where the stem attached one the left side of the grapefruit.

- Cut down from the midpoint of the top.

Oranges

To cut sections from an orange or grapefruit:

- Position the scar where the stem attached on the left side.

- Slice down vertically about 1/2" from the left and right sides to remove the top and bottom.

- Stand the fruit up on one cut end.

- Cut downward around the outside to remove the rest of the peel. Turn the fruit over and work from both ends.

- Cut inward towards the center axis on either side of the membranes to free the segments.

Chapter 11

Practical Tips

Practical tips for making and sustaining changes in your eating pattern including: general guidelines, eat this/not that alternatives to favorite foods, tips for eating away from home and frequently asked questions.

General Guidelines

Collected advice for dealing with a range of issues.

Ten Rules

Ten rules for healthy living [156]:

1. Avoid fast food
   Fast food contributes to weight gain and health problems. Avoid it completely during the first six weeks of changing your eating pattern. If there is no alternative, select the best available options (see "Eating Away from Home" on page 210).

2. Drink water
   Liquid calories may not fill you up but they certainly add up. Put soft drinks, juices, sodas and diet sodas out of bounds. When you are thirsty, drink water, with lemon, lime or orange slices if you prefer.

3. Eat salads
   Mixed greens are loaded with nutrients and have almost no calories. Including green salad with just a tablespoon or two of dressing or oil

and vinegar at the start of every dinner will help fill you up so you eat less overall.

4. Get some exercise every day
Begin with at least 20 minutes of any exercise, even walking, if you can. Make it a rule to do it no less than five days a week.

5. Make sleep a priority
You will have more control over your appetite and more energy for exercise if you sleep soundly. Commit to a consistent eight hours per night, if possible.

6. Mind your mouth
Avoid mindless eating and eat only when eating is your primary activity. Munching while doing something else leads to eating amnesia, eating way too much of the wrong foods without realizing it.

7. Eat foods with identifiable ingredients
Avoid foods with unpronounceable ingredients or you may end up consuming additives and chemicals with little or no nutritional value. With real foods, you know what the ingredients are.

8. Plan all eating occasions
Go off the 'see food' diet and eat only what you intend to eat, when you intend to eat it. Just because food appears, like cake at the office, does not mean you should eat it. Eat when you are hungry and stop when you have had enough—before you are feeling full.

9. Tell everyone
Let the most important people in your life know what health-related changes you want to make and why. Tell them about these rules so they can help you stick to them.

10. Choose what you chew
Take control of your food choices at home and away. Take wholesome foods with you so you always have them available.

Stay on Schedule

Sticking to a regular schedule for meals and sleep is better for your health. Healthy eating is easier when the time between meals is predictable and comfortable.

Staying on a schedule will help you avoid overeating traps like:

- I am not going to eat again for hours so I should fuel up now to carry me over.

- It has been hours since I last ate, I must eat (or I deserve to eat) everything or anything.

- Eating shortly before bed, which interferes with restful sleep and increases fat accumulation. Not sleeping well, or not getting enough sleep, can make you eat more than normal the next day.

After you have been following our recommended eating pattern for a few weeks, you may notice that your appetite changes and it takes longer for you to become hungry after a meal. Your energy level may also be consistent higher and less likely to fade when you have not eaten recently.

Try these ideas if a meal is delayed:

- Drink some water, this will help you feel more energetic and keep your stomach from growling. Tea and coffee are also options but be careful about excessive caffeine.

- Use healthy snacks like nuts to tide you over, if needed, but think of the snack as part of the delayed meal and eat less at that meal.

Research shows that fasting for 12-16 hours overnight improves blood glucose regulation and may thereby reduce the risk of diabetes and cancer [157]. Reducing food intake between 5 PM and midnight and fasting for longer nightly intervals (diurnal cycle) may reduce systemic inflammation and disease risk [158].

Arrange your schedule to take advantage of these effects, if you can:

- Eat breakfast before noon for better all day glucose regulation. Skipping breakfast can result in higher blood glucose after lunch and dinner [159].

- Have your evening meal early, ideally before 6 PM.

- Make the evening meal relatively small, less than 30% of daily calories.

- Brush your teeth after dinner and do not eat again until breakfast.

Changing Your Tastes

Foods high in fat, sugar, and flour are highly rewarding and trigger biological signals that make you crave similar foods. Changing your tastes and breaking free of this cycle can be almost like dealing with drug addiction.

The bad news: your best option may be to quit these foods cold turkey and go through withdrawal. The good news: it only takes a few days for your tastes to change, you are likely to feel much better, and the process does not include the physical pain of drug withdrawal. Some people feel fuzzyheaded or irritable briefly during the transition but nothing serious.

Eat Mindfully

Make mealtime device free. Turn off the television and put away your phone or other devices.

Take a moment to focus before you eat. Say grace, meditate, or just have a calming drink of water as you prepare to enjoy your meal.

Eat mindfully. Pay attention to your food and savor each mouthful. Eat slowly and deliberately. Set your fork down between bites.

Ideally, conversations over meals should be pleasant and relaxed. If the conversation becomes intense or demanding, arrange a time-out until you finish eating. Lingering to talk at the table after a meal can be very pleasant but move any extra food out of reach and sight to limit temptation.

Avoid eating while engaged in any other activity and you will be less likely to eat 'automatically' while distracted by something else. If you must snack while doing something else, take a small serving and keep the rest of the food in another room where you cannot see it or reach it.

Smaller Plates

Use smaller plates and glasses so your serving looks larger. Smaller serving utensils also help.

Avoid eating from a large container because you are likely to eat more. Where you can, buy foods in smaller packages instead of the 55-gallon Costco special. Seeing a large quantity of food actually makes you likely to eat more.

Measure Serving Sizes

"Clever people and grocers, they weigh everything." Zorba the Greek

Estimating a serving size is one of the important skills you may be learning during this process. If you start by measuring servings, you will gradually improve your ability to estimate serving sizes visually without measuring.

A small electronic scale makes it easy to measure serving sizes for many foods. Look for one with features for automatically adjusting for the weight of a dish (tare) and the ability to switch between ounces and grams.

You can also learn to estimate volumes by comparing to the size of common items. For example:

- 1 cup is about the size of a tennis ball or an average woman's fist

- 3-4 ounces of cooked meat: the size of your palm or a deck of playing cards

- 1 ounce of cheese is the size of 2 dominoes,

Out-of-Sight, Out-of-Mind

If you have any foods on our Eat Rarely or Never list at home or work, keep them out of sight. Store them in a place that is hard to access to avoid being tempted by seeing them frequently or being able to get at them easily.

Arrange things so you see healthier options from our Eat Primarily list before you get to the less desirable foods.

Best Way to Cheat

At least during your first few months following this eating plan, if you going to eat something on the Eat Rarely or Never list do it away from home. This will make it easier to stick with your new eating pattern while you are at home.

You may also feel better if you space foods on the Eat Rarely or Never list out over time. For example, only have these foods as part of one meal per day and avoid eating these foods on consecutive days.

Parenting Tips

Primary lymphedema and lipedema are inheritable conditions. Here are some suggestions if you are planning, expecting, or raising an infant with a family history of either condition:

- Seek personalized advice on prenatal nutrition from a registered dietitian. Some women with lipedema gain 100 pounds or more during pregnancy.

- Supplement doses may need to be adjusted for weight changes during pregnancy.

- Ask your health care provider about planning to inoculate the baby with birth-canal bacteria following delivery via caesarean section. Initial findings suggest this establishes a personal microbiota more similar to the microbiota of babies born vaginally, which may have long-term health benefits.

- Breast-feed for at least several weeks, if possible.

- Avoid soy-based infant formula out of concern about the quantity of plant-based estrogens.

- Minimize high fructose juices such as apple juice.

Children at risk or diagnosed with these conditions should follow our recommended eating pattern with appropriate foods and snacks. Young children are more sensitive to the taste of dark green leafy vegetables; blanched or cooked vegetables will be more acceptable. See Appendix E for books with recipes suitable for children.

Trouble Sleeping

In general, following our recommended eating pattern will help you feel better and improve sleep issues. However, there may be some exceptions. Tracking your sleep along with a food diary can help you resolve these issues.

Things to look for if you have trouble sleeping as you change your eating pattern:

- When are you having caffeine in coffee, tea, colas, certain other sodas, 'energy drinks', chocolate, or foods (like tealeaf salad)? Caffeine can take 6-8 hours to wear off and should be limited to early in the day.

- An alcoholic "nightcap" might help you get to sleep, but alcohol keeps you in lighter stages of sleep (not deep sleep or REM sleep) and you may wake up when the alcohol wears off during the night.

- A light snack before bed is okay (if you really need it), but a large meal can cause indigestion that interferes with sleep. Drinking too much in the evening can cause frequent awakenings to urinate.

- Are you getting enough to eat or are you getting hungry during the night?

- Do you need some carbohydrate as part of your evening meal? High protein/low carb meals can sometimes interfere with sleep.

- Gas and cramps at night? Use your food diaries to look for patterns; you may be sensitive to high-fructose foods or other types of foods.

If you have trouble sleeping several nights a week, talk to your health care provider. There are effective treatments including cognitive-behavioral therapy for insomnia.

Eat This/Not That

Quick guide to changes for more health promoting foods.

- Bacon: veggie bacon products made with tempeh.

- Baked beans: most canned products are very sweet and have too much sauce; try mixing baked beans with plain navy beans to cut the sweetness, or make your own sauce. Chili beans are a more savory alternative.

- Baked potato: instead of starchy Russet or Idaho potatoes, try baking sweet potato or yam, or roasting smaller waxy varieties such as red potatoes, Yukon or gold potatoes, purple potatoes, etc. Top with a little kefir, yogurt or butter instead of sour cream.

- Barbeque: chopped tempeh sloppy joe or tempeh strips with home-made or low-sodium barbeque sauce.

- Beer: gluten free beer and hard cider are options you can try. These products vary greatly in terms of taste and nutritional desirability.

- Birthday cake: see our recipe for "Almond Cake" on page 175.

- Burgers: try grilled Portobello mushrooms, veggie burgers made from beans, vegetables, or tofu, tempeh or tofu cut to burger size. Use plenty of caramelized onions, mushrooms, sautéed peppers, and other plant-based toppings, plus your favorite condiments.

- Candy: try smaller candies with intense flavors such as mints, or crystalized ginger, and savor the taste rather than chomping a handful.

- Cereal: oatmeal, granola (not too sweet), other whole grain and gluten free options.

- Chicken breast: try smaller servings of breast meat or chicken thighs, which are smaller, tastier, and contain nutrients found only in dark meat.

- Chips: baked corn chips that are lightly salted.

- Chocolate: small amounts of dark chocolate with at least 70% cacao.

- Cream cheese: smaller amount of cream cheese, Neufchatel, goat cheese, thick Greek yogurt, hummus, or bean spread.

- Cream or coffee whiteners: cow milk or almond milk.

- Crema (Mexican topping): yogurt with a little salt added.

- Dessert: have just a small amount, taste pie filling but not crust or topping,

- Dips: replace sour cream-based or packaged dips with homemade dips, see "Dips or Spreads" on page 185.

- Food bars or protein bars: package up single servings of nuts, trail mix, granola, etc.

- French fries: bake wedges of sweet potato, yam, or smaller varieties of potatoes brushed with a little olive oil. Add a little salt at the table.

- Hot dogs: try meat alternative hot dogs; use good mustard and naturally fermented sauerkraut.

- Ice cream: coconut ice cream in limited amounts.

- Lettuce: iceberg and other light green lettuces only provide a few nutrients. Try arugula, romaine, baby kale, spinach, and other dark green alternatives.

- Lunchmeats: try veggie meat products, sliced tempeh or tofu; use tasty mustard or other condiments.

- Mashed potatoes: real mashed potatoes made with smaller waxy potatoes are good; avoid instant potato products and Russet/Idaho potatoes. Try leaving skins on, adding garlic or horseradish for flavor, or mashing potatoes and cauliflower together for a lower carb version.

- Matzo and matzo balls: if you can eat gluten safely, have a small serving of wheat-based matzo and matzo balls; if not, look for gluten free recipes or have small amounts of gluten-free products.

- Pastries: have a fraction of a pastry or have berries, fruit or a toasted corn tortilla.

- Pie: taste the filling without the crust or topping.

- Pizza: make your own pizza using flatbreads or tortillas, caramelized onions, sautéed peppers, and other vegetable toppings.

- Red meats: try smaller servings of more flavorful cuts, think of meat as a flavor accent rather than the main attraction, try meat substitutes (see "Meat Substitutes" on page 143).

- Snacks: nuts, dried berries or fruit. See "Light Snacks" on page 140.

- Soda/pop: replace sweetened beverages (regular or diet) with water (add lemon, lime or orange for flavor), unsweetened tea, coconut water (unsweetened), or other healthy drinks.

- Sour cream: replace with plain yogurt or kefir.

- Spaghetti: try steamed spaghetti squash strands or black bean pasta as alternatives to wheat. See "Pasta Alternatives" on page 142.

- Turkey stuffing: try stuffing based on brown rice or wild rice in place of bread or make stuffing using gluten-free cornbread (made with less sugar).

- Whipped cream: try plain kefir on berries or desserts.

- White rice: brown rice, oatmeal, or quinoa.

- White wine: try tasting different red wines, rosé, or red wine with a little water.

Eating Away from Home

Tips for finding recommended foods in restaurants or convenience stores, selecting foods at a buffet or potluck, and air travel.

Restaurants

Finding vegetables and complex carbohydrates without gluten or excess salt at restaurants can be a tricky but is doable. Vegetarian and gluten-free offerings may be available that are not on the regular menu, so ask.

Looking online can make the process easier because many restaurants post nutritional information on their websites. You can also can find reviews, menus, and ratings in online guides.

Healthy Dining Finder (www.healthydiningfinder.com) can help you select better menu choices at some popular restaurants by setting the personalized search options. Review these recommendations carefully to locate options that are truly are suitable for you.

Here are ordering suggestions for different types of restaurants:

- Barbeque: beans, greens, coleslaw, salads, meats with 'dry rub' spices, etc. Limit sauces high in sugar and salt and avoid fried foods, breads, sweets.

- Breakfast, Pancake or Waffle Places: vegetable omelet (not mixed with pancake batter), salads, vegetable side dishes, eggs, grilled potatoes, etc. Avoid fatty meats, fried foods, breads, pancakes, waffles, syrups, and sweets.

- Burger Places: salads, coleslaw, vegetable side dishes, order burgers without bun (if you eat beef); avoid bread products, fried foods, and sweets. Veggie burgers made from beans and vegetables are OK but many are primarily rice or tofu.

- Chinese: soups, lots of vegetable options, lettuce wraps, fish, seafood, lean meats, etc. Have a small amount of brown rice, order plain steamed vegetables or less sauce than usual; stay away from sweet sauces, noodle products (high salt and gluten), anything deep-fried, sweets.

- Coffee shop: coffee, fruit, nuts, oatmeal (unsweetened), salads, tea, yogurt; not pastries, sweet drinks, sweets.

- French: salads, soups, vegetables, seafood, meats; limit rich sauces and cheeses; avoid breads, pasta, fried foods, and sweets.

- Greek and Middle Eastern: salads, lentil soup, vegetable dishes, hummus, baba ganoush (eggplant dip), seafood, lamb and other meats, etc. Limit the rice and deep fried falafel; avoid the pita bread, tabbouleh, gyros meat, and sweets.

- Indian: lentil dahl, garbanzo beans (chana masala), spinach (palak paneer), vegetable dishes, curries, yogurt (raita), etc. Limit brown rice and avoid naan, fried appetizers, sweets, etc.

- Italian: look for soup, salads, marinated vegetables (antipasto), spinach and other vegetable side dishes, grilled seafood or meats, etc. Stay away from bread, breadsticks, pasta, breaded or fried foods, sweets, etc.

- Japanese: salads, pickles, sashimi, miso soup, spinach and other vegetable dishes, pickled ginger, tofu, natto, etc. Limit rice, especially sweetened sushi rice and inari sushi; avoid salty sauces, noodle products, tempura and other fried foods.

- Mexican: salads, soups, guacamole, salsa, black beans or whole pinto beans, corn tortillas, baked chips, etc. Limit white rice, grilled meats; avoid cheese, sour cream (Mexican crema), refried beans (made with lard), wheat tortillas, anything fried, sweets, etc.

- Pizza: soup, salads and vegetable side dishes. Avoid the pizza, bread products, pasta, and sweets.

- Salad bars: salad, vegetables, beans, etc. Avoid bread, croutons, and sweets.

- Seafood: healthy seafood, salads, vegetables. Avoid breads, fried foods, and sweets.

- Steak houses: soup, salads, vegetable side dishes (without cream). Limit grilled meats, rice, rich or salty sauces; avoid bread, baked potatoes, fried foods, sweets, etc.

- Thai: salads, vegetable dishes, coconut milk curries, seafood, meats; limit brown rice, avoid fried foods, noodles, sweet or salty sauces, and sweets.

Buffets and Potlucks

Look at the whole buffet first to see what food choices are available, and then decide what you want to eat. Avoid the trap of 'discovering' things you 'just have to try.'

Choose a seat where you cannot see the food. Resist the temptation to go back for get more food, just because you can.

If you have trouble limiting what you eat, eat somewhere else or pass up the buffet.

Convenience Stores

Many convenience foods are high in sugar, fat, salt or gluten. Here are the better choices:

- Fruit: apple, banana, orange,

- Hard-boiled eggs

- Hummus

- Nuts or seeds without salt or sugar

- Salads: green salad, bean salad, coleslaw, etc. Use small amounts of salad dressing and avoid salty cheeses and croutons.

- Tuna or tuna salad

- Vegetable sticks or appetizers: baby carrots, broccoli, celery, cherry tomatoes, etc.

- Water, unsweetened tea, orange juice

- Yogurt, plain unsweetened if available or 'fruit at the bottom' and leave the fruit

Air Travel

Avoid salt and stay well hydrated before, during, and after flying to minimize swelling:

- Drink water, orange juice, water with a splash of orange juice, or unsweetened tea. Limit coffee to your normal amount and avoid sweetened drinks, fruit juices (other than orange juice), and high-salt tomato juice drinks.

- Bring healthy snacks like plain nuts and vegetable sticks, if you want them. Pass up any cookies, crackers, nuts with salt or sugar, salty snacks, or sweets.

- Plan on bringing food from home or shopping in the airport for healthier options. Solid foods and up to 3.4 ounces (100 ml) of liquid (such as yogurt) are allowed through airport security, per TSA rules.

Frequently Asked Questions

Can I have chocolate?

Yes, dark chocolate with at least 70% cacao is best, in small servings.

Do I have to give up sweets?

No but you may want to limit sweets in terms of quantity and frequency. You may also notice that your tastes change, your craving for refined sweets fades away, and you prefer berries and fruits.

Do I have to give up my favorite food?

This depends on your specific health issues. If you have celiac disease, food allergies, or a similar condition, and your favorite food can trigger your condition, you will feel better if you strictly avoid that food.

If you can safely eat your favorite food but it appears on our Eat Rarely or Never list, try eating it in smaller quantities and less often.

Should I stop eating animal products?

This is up to you, and may depend on your health concerns. Research shows health benefits from eating less meat but some people find it hard to give up animal foods for a variety of reasons. Linda-Anne (our lipedema exemplar) does not eat meat (other than fish), has very little dairy, and does eat eggs.

How much fat should I eat?

Benefits from limiting fat depend upon your health concerns. To prevent or reverse heart disease (including congestive heart failure) or if you are concerned about fatty liver disease, plan to eat very little fat and no animal products. Lymphedema and lipedema will benefit from similar limits.

Must I give up bread/gluten?

Reactions to gluten vary widely and have far-reaching health effects. We recommend an initial gluten free period because this helps people see if they feel better without gluten, and helps correct gut dysbiosis. After being gluten free for several months, keep a food diary while you reintroduce whole grain wheat and see how you feel.

Bread with less gluten is an option while transitioning to gluten-free or for longer-term use. For example, Ezekiel brand multigrain breads.

Do I have to cook?

Making mindful decisions about what to eat is the most important thing. Everyone has options for wise food choices. Food choices do not need be perfect in order to be better, in terms of your health.

If you cook, or have someone who will cook for you, you gain more control over what you eat and have more options. You can follow our recommended eating plan while eating out, getting take-out, or prepared foods. How easily you can do this will depend upon the food options in your area.

Are spices OK?

Yes, herbs and spices have health promoting properties and can be used as liberally as you like. Check the sodium content of spice mixtures.

What can I do about gas?

Some digestive gas is normal with this eating pattern because fiber is fermented in the gut, which produces gas as well as beneficial short-chain fatty acids. You may have more gas than usual during the first few weeks as your gut microbiota adjusts to processing different types of foods.

If gas is a persistent problem, keep a food diary to identify the specific foods that give you gas or other digestive issues. Foods known to contain FODMAP compounds are likely suspects and are identified in the shopping guide in Appendix A.

If beans are causing gas, be sure fresh or dried beans are cooked completely before tasting or serving them. Try other varieties of beans, some people are fine with small beans but not large beans like kidney beans. If beans are a trigger, you can try a specific enzyme supplement, such as Beano.

Why do these greens taste bitter?

Many vegetables have a bitter taste from chemicals that keep predators from eating them, which are the same chemicals that help fight disease. You can make greens taste better by cooking them lightly (not too little or too much) and serving them with a little fat (oil, butter, or nuts) or other flavors, such as garlic or tomato.

Children are more sensitive to these tastes than adults are which is why they may balk at eating greens. Blanching vegetables will help sweeten up the taste and make vegetables more acceptable.

Where can I find more recipes?

Look online to find recipes for plant-based and gluten-free versions of your favorite foods or things you can make using Eat Primarily ingredients.

Where is the best place to shop for ingredients?

Shop where you get a good selection, especially of fresh foods. Farmers markets and ethnic markets are great. You may be able to find seasonal deals at dollar stores or big discount stores. Beware of free tastings and samples in retail stores; these are usually highly processed foods.

Can I have recommended ingredients delivered?

There are local grocery delivery services in many areas that offer fresh and frozen foods, as well as other grocery store items. Many small markets will provide local delivery service if you ask.

Big online retailers offer a very wide range of food products and specialty foods. Check shipping costs, especially if you order anything perishable or frozen.

Community supported agriculture (CSA) is another option where you subscribe for periodic deliveries of fresh produce from local farmers. Look online for CSA directories such as Local Harvest (www.localharvest.org) or the USDA local food directory (www.ams.usda.gov).

Should I grow my own food?

If it is practical for you to grow your own vegetables, fruit, chickens, or other animals, it can provide many benefits in terms of food freshness and flavor. Working with soil and live animals also increases the healthy diversity of gut microbes. Even growing fresh herbs in a window box helps.

Will this food cost more?

Food costs are generally similar for whole foods and plant based, with fewer animal products, compared to conventional eating patterns. If food does cost more, consider it an investment in your health.

If you are eating at home, your cost of groceries will probably be comparable or less than current costs. This includes spending less on processed foods and animal products and more on produce, including organic produce. Food costs may very more during the year, especially if you buy expensive out of season produce.

When eating out or getting take-out, plant based entrées are generally less expensive than meat-based entrees. You may also save on beverages and desserts.

Preparing foods at home can be significantly less expensive than eating out, take out, or fast food. Gluten-free foods (or gluten substitute foods) and meat alternatives are expensive but we recommend minimizing them based on their nutritional properties, not their cost.

What are some good cheap eats?

Plant based foods provide much more cost-effective nutrition than animal products or processed foods. Here are some low cost food ideas:

- Vegetables and fruits that are in season or on special.

- Beans and brown rice are inexpensive sources of carbohydrate and protein.

- Sweet potatoes and yams.

- Cabbage: red and green cabbage provide many nutrients and keep well.

- Onions and garlic.

You can save money by spending time preparing foods instead of buying convenience foods. For example, dried beans cost less than canned or frozen beans; cooking brown rice is less expensive than ready-to-eat rice or take-out. Be sure to soak dried kidney beans for at least 5 hours, change the water, and boil them for at least 10 minutes before eating (or tasting).

Larger packages are less expensive, in terms of cost per serving, if you can manage them. Look for places that sell the larger 'food service' size cans and packages.

Foods that are sold in bulk are generally less expensive (your mileage may vary) and provide the convenience of only buying as much as you need.

What equipment do I need?

Basic cooking equipment for one or two people and small groups:

- Small frying pan

- Medium frying pan (10") with a lid
- Large frying pan (12") with a lid: use for larger quantities or foods, such as squash or potatoes, which need contact with the pan to cook.
- Wok or stir-fry pan with a lid (12")
- Small saucepan
- Medium saucepan
- Pot with a lid: for making soups or large dishes
- Colander: for rinsing or draining foods
- Baking dish: 8x8 inch glass
- Baking sheets, baking pans, or cookie sheets: one or more
- Chef's knife with a wide, curved, blade and a comfortable grip. A wide blade keeps your knuckles off the cutting board while chopping and can be used to scoop up chopped foods.
- Utility knife for smaller tasks
- Spatula
- Cooking spoons: regular, slotted
- Cutting boards: portable boards are easier to clean than built-in.
- Potholders or hot mitts
- Measuring cups and spoons
- Grater
- Colander
- Blender: high power blender or food processor: optional, only required for smoothies.

Any cooking tips?

Lessons learned from experience:

- Work with two cutting boards, one for initial trimming and food scraps, the other for final chopping and ready-to-use foods. This makes it easier to transfer foods to the pan or serving dish.

- Wear a protective cut resistant glove if you need one, especially if you are at risk of lymphedema in your hand and arm. Cut resistant gloves for cooking are available online or at restaurant supply stores.

- Be cautious about multi-tasking. Turn burners off if you are interrupted, or something takes longer than expected.

- Err on the side of undercooking for dishes without animal products, undercooked vegetables taste better than overcooked. Dishes containing eggs or meats are safer if fully cooked.

- Some people overlap preparing ingredients and cooking while others prefer to have everything prepped before starting to cook. This is a personal preference; use the approach that make you most comfortable.

Chapter **12:**

Record Keeping

Routine records are recommended for anyone with, or at risk for, lymphedema or lipedema. Record keeping serves multiple purposes and the types of records you need will change over time, depending on what is going on. You cannot rely only on the records kept by your health care provider because they may not learn of minor changes in your condition.

The types of records described below and their functions include:

- Weight records help monitor your condition and can help with problem solving many issues. We recommend tracking weight daily while changing your eating pattern, changing medications or supplements, or when anything unusual is going on medically; weekly records are OK at other times.

- Foods and Moods records are intended to help you change your eating pattern. Continuing these records after you have established new habits is optional.

- Food Diaries (all varieties) are troubleshooting tools for food-related issues and only need to be kept as needed.

- Activity Tracking is also a tool for changing behaviors and is optional after new habits have been established.

- Limb Measurements help monitor your condition and help protect against ill-fitting compression garments. Most people should track measurements at least weekly on an ongoing basis.

- Body Temperature should be measured to establish a baseline and monitored, as needed, if you think you may have an infection.

Some people keep their records private while others share records online where family and friends can see their progress and provide support and encouragement. Another option is to display your records where you will see them and be reminded of your goals at times when you look for food. For example, on the refrigerator door.

Records are essential for reinforcement (see "Create Reinforcements" on page 115) during the process of building new habits. If you are using reinforcement, set up your records to show each of the reinforcement dates and events so that you can see your progress and each step toward your goal.

Weight

Tracking your weight on a daily basis provides an important tool for monitoring your lymphedema and overall health, especially if you have congestive heart failure or chronic venous insufficiency.

Changes in swelling or water retention clearly affect your weight because water and tissue fluid are dense and the amount of fluid can change quickly. Changes in body fat or muscle mass are harder to detect because these are less dense and change more gradually.

Weigh yourself at the same time every day in similar clothing. First thing in the morning (after toileting) is good. Consistent time of day is important because some people (especially women with lipedema) gain weight during the day. Women with lipedema may fluctuate several pounds from one day to the next, depending on activity levels and food intake.

Women who are menstruating should also track the date when their period starts and day number within each cycle. Many women routinely gain and lose weight during their cycles. For these women, it may be more meaningful to compare weights to the same day number of previous cycles, than to compare today to yesterday or the day before. For example, if your cycle is 28 days you would compare today to 28 days ago (previous cycle) and 56 days ago (cycle before that).

If you have trouble seeing or reading a scale, look for a digital scale with options such as a remote display you can mount at eye level, digital memory, or ability to send readings your smartphone app or PC via a wireless interface

Form 12-1: Weight Record

Name:							Week of:	
	M	T	W	T	F	S	S	
Previous Weight								
Weight								
Weight Change								
Measurements								
Day of Cycle								
Notes								

(Wi-Fi or Bluetooth). Scales are also available for extended weight ranges (bariatric scales).

You can track your weight on paper, in a smartphone app (such as Apple Health or Google Fit), or a spreadsheet.

Along with weight, you may want to note:

- Changes in types or dosages of medications or supplements.

- Infections or other health events.

- Changes in eating pattern or foods. For example, if you are experimenting.

Foods and Moods

The Foods and Moods record provides a simple way of tracking how you are doing in terms of food choices and overall energy level. Use this to track your progress and identify when you need to look in more detail. You can track this on paper, using a smartphone app, or a spreadsheet (such as Apple Numbers or Microsoft Excel).

Update the Foods and Moods Record throughout the day:

- First thing in the morning, enter your weight. See the instructions for weight given above.

- Each time you eat or drink anything other than water, unsweetened coffee or tea, rate what you ate based on the lists in Chapter 3 Recommended Eating Pattern: 1) mostly Eat Primarily foods, 2) mostly Eat Occasionally Foods, or 3) mostly Eat Rarely or Never foods.

- Also record why you are eating. For example, are you eating because you are hungry, it is mealtime, or because you are bored, seeking comfort, want to reward yourself, or for other reasons?

- At the end of the day, rate your overall mood and energy for the day on a scale of 1) Very Good to 5) Not Good; enter the total of your meal ratings and (optionally) fill in the day number of your menstrual cycle. Note positive events or achievements for the day or negatives.

If your records show that you are eating for emotional reasons or eating unusual quantities (either small or large), see "Overcoming Emotional Is-

Form 12-2: Foods and Moods Record

Name:		Week of:						
		M	T	W	T	F	S	S
Breakfast	Rating							
	Why							
AM Snack(s)	Rating							
	Why							
Lunch	Rating							
	Why							
PM Snack(s)	Rating							
	Why							
Dinner	Rating							
	Why							
Evening Snack(s)	Rating							
	Why							
Meal Ratings Total								
Mood Rating (1-5)								
Energy Rating (1-5)								
Notes								

sues" on page 123.

Food Diary

A food diary tracks what foods you ate and the quantity of each food. If you are working with a dietitian, ask them about keeping a food diary and what tools they can offer.

There are several options with different levels of detail, as explained below:

- Basic Food Diary tracks foods and quantities without nutritional information. This can be a paper process and is useful for monitoring and experimentation.

- Carbohydrate Counting tracks only carbohydrates and can be useful for establishing and maintaining a regular eating pattern. This can be a paper process or use computerized tools.

- Nutritional Analysis systems look at foods in terms of multiple nutrients and provide many additional capabilities.

If your records show that you are eating unusual quantities (either small or large), see "Overcoming Emotional Issues" on page 123.

Basic Food Diary

A basic food diary records foods and quantities in a form that is convenient and meaningful for you. This can be paper, smartphone notes, or online note taking tools. You may also want to record where you are eating, if you are away from home.

Carbohydrate Counting

Carbohydrate counting uses the net carbohydrate content (also known as available carbohydrate) of foods calculated as Total Carbohydrate minus Fiber. You can do this manually using information from nutrition labels, 'food count' books (such as Calorie King or Nutribase), online food databases and recipe calculators, or smartphone apps. There are also apps and online services for tracking carb intake.

People with diabetes use a similar method to plan their carbohydrate intake or determine how much insulin they need. Diabetics sometimes use 'carb units' equal to 15g of net carbohydrate.

Nutritional Analysis

Nutritional analysis takes information on foods eaten and calculates quantities of nutrients contained in these foods, and (optionally) may compare intake to recommended daily values. Some systems have detailed databases with information on a large number of foods and nutrients including menu items from popular restaurants. Some smartphone apps can scan a product bar code and instantly retrieve nutritional information.

This level of detail can be very helpful for identifying issues and improving your eating pattern. If you have a lot of variety in what you eat, the record keeping can be time-consuming, even with automated tools, and you may only want to do it occasionally.

Computerized food diary tools make it easier to get a detailed nutritional analysis of what you are eating and these tools can help you:

- Calculate your baseline calorie requirements based on your resting metabolic rate and typical activity level.

- Establish goals for changing your weight, translate these goals into calorie targets, and track your progress.

- Compare what you are eating to your target values for calories and nutrients.

- Evaluate calories used by various activities that you are tracking.

For example:

- My Net Diary offers a variety of smartphone apps and online systems for food and activity tracking for a monthly fee, following a free trial period. The service can share data with fitness trackers and electronic scales. See www.mynetdiary.com.

- Super Tracker free online tools from the USDA provide the ability to track and analyze food intake, evaluate physical activity and support the process of setting and reaching goals. Caution: Super Tracker uses calorie patterns from the IOM Dietary Guidelines for Americans 2010 that are higher carbohydrate than our recommendations and the calorie patterns for 1,400 calories/day or less are only for children under the age of nine. See www.supertracker.usda.gov.

Activity Tracking

Track daily activity and exercise in a way that is meaningful for you and will help you see changes. There are many ways to do this including:

- Smartphone apps such as Apple Health or Google Fit can measure things like steps, distance walked, flights of stairs climbed, etc. Note that you must wear or carry your phone to get these measurements.

- Personal fitness monitors such as Apple Watch, Fitbit, Jawbone Up, or Nike Fuel Band provide activity tracking without requiring that you wear your phone. Some devices can also measure sleep time and movement.

- Pedometers are simple, less expensive alternatives to high tech monitors.

- Measuring or estimating number of minutes spent exercising or even just moving around with a timer or watch.

Limb Measurements

Tracking limb measurements provides useful information for managing lymphedema or lipedema. Measurement in one or two places per limb is faster and easier than the more detailed measurements made by a therapist or fitter.

Note: procedures are provided for arm and leg measurements only. Check with your lymphedema therapist about measuring other affected body parts.

Measurements can help you:

- Identify any changes in limb size that could indicate an infection or other issue.

- Be sure your compression garments fit properly. Compression garments that are too tight can be harmful and garments that are too loose are not protective or beneficial.

Therapists measure in centimeters (even in the US). Ask your lymphedema therapist where you can get a fitter's tape measure. If you are using a ruler marked in inches, the conversion factor is 1" = 2.54 cm.

You will need the following equipment:

- A cloth tape measure or a specialized tape measure sold by lymphedema supply companies.

- A washable marker, ballpoint pen, or eyebrow pencil for marking positions.

- A calculator for comparing past and present measurement values.

Measurement guidelines:

- Measure at the same time of day (morning is best) without compression.

- Have your limb be in the same position every time.

- Be consistent about how you position the tape and take the measurement.

Measurement locations for arms and legs are given in the sidebars on page 230 and page 231.

Body Temperature

Measure body temperature using a thermometer in the mouth (oral), ear, rectum, or under the armpit. Always use the same measurement location for comparable results.

Check your temperature periodically to establish a baseline. Many people have normal temperatures that are less than 98.6°F and for some people a reading of 98.6°F indicates a slight fever.

Check your temperature any time you suspect you may have an infection or fever. If you are not feeling well but there are no objective symptoms of an infection, check your temperature at least every four hours while you are awake.

Contact your health care provider if your oral temperature is more than 100°F (37.8°C) or 2°F (1.1°C) above your baseline temperature. Older people may have a small temperature increase from an infection and children have larger variations.

Leg Measurement Locations

For the leg (see Figure 12-1: Leg Measurements):

- Measure the ankle.

- Measure the largest part of the calf.

- Measure the mid-point of the thigh.

Figure 12-1: Leg Measurements

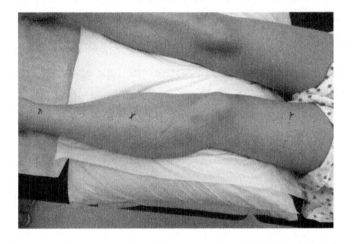

Arm Measurement Locations

For the arm (see Figure 12-2: Arm Measurements):

- Measure the midpoint of the forearm.

- Measure the midpoint of the upper arm.

Figure 12-2: Arm Measurements

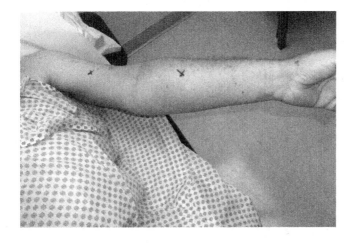

Shopping Guide

Use this guide to select health-promoting foods. We have included a wide variety of foods you may consider trying, according to your tastes. Try a few new foods at a time.

The guide include items to consider in each department of the grocery store. Use it together with the list of packaged and processed foods ingredients to avoid in Appendix B.

Suggestions:

• Shop with a list, at least until you have established a routine. A list makes shopping easier and reduces frustration.

• Avoid shopping when you are hungry or fatigued, if possible. It may be harder to make wise decisions under those conditions.

• Keep a shopping list in your kitchen so you can add items to the list when you use something up, or notice a need.

• Before shopping, review your plans for the next few days to be sure your list includes any foods you need for the meals you are planning.

Area	Foods	Eat	Note
Fresh Vegetables			
Choose organic vegetables, if available, from all parts of the color spectrum.			
	Arugula or salad rocket	Primarily	
	Artichoke (globe)	Primarily	FODMAP, Inulin
	Asparagus	Primarily	FODMAP, Inulin
	Beans (shelled, seed only): cranberry beans, fava beans, garbanzo beans, lima beans, etc.	Primarily	FODMAP
	Beans (whole): Italian or Romano beans, snap beans, string beans, wax beans, etc.	Primarily	
	Chicory greens: Belgian endive, curly endive, escarole, frisee, radicchio, red treviso, salsify	Primarily	FODMAP, Inulin
	Beets and beet leaves	Primarily	
	Broccoli, Chinese broccoli, broccoli rabe or rapini	Primarily	
	Brussels sprouts	Primarily	
	Cabbage: green and red, Napa cabbage/Chinese cabbage, Savoy cabbage	Primarily	
	Carrots	Primarily	
	Cauliflower: white, green, orange, purple	Primarily	FODMAP
	Celeriac/celery root	Primarily	
	Celery	Primarily	FODMAP
	Corn on the cob	Primarily	
	Dandelion greens	Primarily	FODMAP, Inulin
	Fennel	Primarily	
	Garlic	Primarily	FODMAP, Inulin
	Ginger root/fresh ginger	Primarily	

Area	Foods	Eat	Note
	Greens: bok choy/pak choy, chard/Swiss chard, collards, endive, kale, mustard greens, spinach, turnip greens, etc.	Primarily	
	Herbs: basil, cilantro, mint, oregano, parsley, rosemary, sage, tarragon, thyme, etc.	Primarily	
	Jerusalem artichoke, burdock root, sunchoke, yacon	Primarily	FODMAP, Inulin
	Jicama, Mexican yam bean, or Mexican turnip	Primarily	FODMAP, Inulin
	Kohlrabi, German turnip or turnip cabbage	Primarily	
	Leeks or ramps	Primarily	FODMAP, Inulin
	Lettuce: Boston, butter lettuce, field greens, iceberg, little gem, red lettuce, romaine, spring mix, watercress	Primarily	
	Mushrooms: brown, cremini, enoki, Italian, maitake, oyster, portabella, shiitake, white or button	Primarily	FODMAP
	Okra, ladies' fingers, bhendi, gumbo	Primarily	
	Onions: cipollini, green/scallions, pearl, red, spring, sweet/Vidalia, white, yellow; shallots	Primarily	FODMAP, Inulin
	Peas: English peas, green peas	Primarily	
	Peas: Edible-podded, snap peas, snow peas	Primarily	
	Peppers or Chili Peppers: green, purple, red, yellow, etc. and sweet, mild or hot	Primarily	
	Potatoes: new, purple, red, white, yellow/Yukon. Not high-starch baking potatoes, Idaho, or russet.	Primarily	
	Pumpkin (cooking or baking variety)	Primarily	
	Radish many varieties; daikon	Primarily	
	Soybeans/edamame	Primarily	FODMAP

Area	Foods	Eat	Note
	Sprouts: alfalfa, broccoli, daikon, fenugreek, mung bean, onion, radish, sunflower sprouts	Primarily	
	Squash, winter: acorn, butternut, Hubbard, kabocha (Japanese pumpkin), spaghetti, etc.	Primarily	
	Squash, summer: crookneck, scallop, straight neck, zucchini (courgette, marrow), etc.	Primarily	
	Sweet potato or yam	Primarily	
	Tomatoes	Primarily	
	Root vegetables: parsnip, rutabaga, turnip, etc.	Primarily	

Fresh Fruit

Choose organic fruit, if available.

Area	Foods	Eat	Note
	Apples	Primarily	FODMAP
	Apricots	Primarily	FODMAP
	Avocados	Primarily	FODMAP
	Bananas	Primarily	Inulin
	Berries: blueberries, blackberries, strawberries, raspberries, etc.	Primarily	
	Cherries, sweet or sour/tart	Primarily	FODMAP
	Citrus fruits: grapefruits, lemons, limes, mandarins, oranges, satsumas, tangerines, etc.	Primarily	
	Grapes: black, green, pink, purple, red, yellow	Primarily	
	Kiwi fruit	Primarily	
	Mangoes	Primarily	FODMAP
	Melons: cantaloupe, honeydew, etc.	Primarily	
	Nectarines	Primarily	FODMAP
	Papaya	Primarily	

Area	Foods	Eat	Note
	Peaches	Primarily	FODMAP
	Pears	Primarily	FODMAP
	Pineapple	Primarily	
	Plums	Primarily	FODMAP
	Pomegranates	Primarily	
	Watermelon	Primarily	FODMAP

Dairy Foods

Choose organic dairy products without carrageenan or a lot of added sugar.

	Butter	Limited	
	Cheeses (not processed cheese or cheese spread): made from cow, goat or sheep's milk	Limited	
	Eggs, preferably free range organic or omega-3 eggs	Limited	
	Ghee (clarified butter)	Limited	
	Kefir made from cow or goat's milk, plain unsweetened	Primarily	
	Milk	Limited	FODMAP
	Yogurt: plain unsweetened Greek yogurt	Primarily	

Refrigerated Foods

	Almond milk, unsweetened	Primarily	
	Coconut milk beverage, unsweetened	Primarily	
	Hemp milk, unsweetened	Primarily	
	Horseradish	Limited	
	Hummus Look for a brand or flavor with less sodium.	Primarily	FODMAP
	Kimchi	Primarily	
	Natto fermented soybeans	Primarily	
	Miso fermented soybean paste (check sodium content)	Primarily	

Area	Foods	Eat	Note
	Pickles: dill, kosher, half-sour (new pickles), sour pickles, pickled vegetables, etc.	Primarily	
	Sauerkraut	Primarily	
	Tempeh fermented cake: multi-grain or soy	Primarily	
	Tofu or fermented tofu	Primarily	

Frozen Foods

Organic foods are best. Check entrees and seasoned vegetables for sodium content and undesirable ingredients (see the list of ingredients to avoid in Appendix B).

Area	Foods	Eat	Note
	Beans (seeds): kidney beans, lima beans, etc.	Primarily	FODMAP
	Beans (whole): green beans, Italian/Romano beans, snap beans, string beans, wax beans, etc.	Primarily	
	Berries): blueberries, blackberries, raspberries, strawberries	Primarily	
	Cauliflower	Primarily	FODMAP
	Coconut ice cream (in moderation)	Limited	
	Potatoes: small potatoes like fingerling, red, marble, purple, yellow/Yukon golds, etc. Not starchy russet or Idaho potato products: baked, fries, mashed, shapes, shreds, etc.	Primarily	
	Soybeans (edamame).	Primarily	FODMAP
	Sweet potato or yam without sauce	Primarily	
	Vegetables (non-starchy): asparagus, broccoli, Brussels sprouts, carrots, chard, collard greens, kale, okra, snap peas, spinach, snow peas, squash, etc.	Primarily	
	Vegetables (starchy): corn, peas	Primarily	

Area	Foods	Eat	Note
	Fish and Seafood		
	Choose fresh or frozen to widen your selection.		
	Fish (preferably fresh or frozen wild): see the sidebar "Which Fish?"	Primarily	OMEGA-3
	Meat Department		
	Meats, preferably organic and grass-fed not grain-fed	Limited	
	Poultry, preferably free range organic chicken (without skin), turkey, or duck including legs and thighs (dark meat); try smaller heritage breeds if available.	Limited	

Which Fish?

Fish recommendations based on risk/benefit assessment of omega-3 fats vs. mercury [160]:

- Unlimited consumption: pollock, flounder, shrimp, trout, herring, salmon, canned light tuna, cod (black cod, sablefish, butterfish), Atlantic mackerel, and sardines. Tilapia is low in mercury but there are concerns about food safety with fish farmed in China and certain other countries.

- Twice a week: canned white or albacore tuna, halibut, sea bass, lobster.

- Once a week: tuna steak.

- Avoid eat fish that may be higher in mercury such as shark, swordfish, king mackerel (Atlantic mackerel is OK) and tilefish.

Lean fish contain small amounts of fat. Frozen breaded fish products, fish from fast-food outlets, and gefilte fish have minimal amounts of omega-3 fat.

Area	Foods	Eat	Note
Canned Foods			
Choose no salt added or low-sodium canned foods.			
	Anchovies, anchovy paste	Primarily	OMEGA-3
	Artichokes or artichoke hearts, water packed	Primarily	FODMAP, Inulin
	Beans (seeds), Legumes or Pulses: adzuki beans, black beans, butter beans (gigantes), cannellini beans, chickpeas (garbanzo or ceci beans), fava beans, great northern beans, kidney beans, lentils, lima beans, peas, navy beans, pinto beans, etc.	Primarily	FODMAP
	Beans (whole): green beans, Italian/Romano beans, snap beans, string beans, wax beans, etc.	Primarily	
	Broth or stock: organic vegetable or chicken; check the salt content, even 'low salt' can be high in sodium.	Limited	
	Coconut milk or coconut cream for cooking	Primarily	
	Fruit packed in water or juice without added sugar: mandarin oranges, pineapple (canned pineapple does not provide bromelain enzyme), sour/tart cherries, etc.	Primarily	
	Herring	Primarily	OMEGA-3
	Nut butter made from walnuts, cashews, almonds, or macadamia nuts	Primarily	
	Olives	Primarily	
	Salmon, canned sockeye	Primarily	OMEGA-3
	Sardines packed in water or olive oil	Primarily	OMEGA-3
	Soups: vegetable or bean based, low sodium or no-salt added.	Primarily	

Area	Foods	Eat	Note
	Tomatoes, chopped, crushed, ground, or fire-roasted are best because they include the seeds; tomato paste, tomato puree, tomato sauce, etc. are also good. Preferably low sodium and no added sugars.	Primarily	
	Tuna packed in water	Primarily	OMEGA-3
	Vegetables (non-starchy): asparagus, carrots, collard greens, kale, spinach, snow peas, squash, etc.	Primarily	
	Vegetables (starchy): corn, peas, potatoes, sweet potato or yam, etc.	Primarily	

Dried Beans

Area	Foods	Eat	Note
	Dried Beans (seeds), Legumes or Pulses: dried beans, chickpeas/garbanzo beans, lentils, peas, etc.	Primarily	FODMAP

Grains

Choose naturally gluten-free grains and whole-grain products. Avoid grains containing gluten (all varieties of wheat, rye, barley) and gluten-free products made from rice, potato starch, tapioca, etc.

Area	Foods	Eat	Note
	Cereals that are gluten-free, not rice-based, and not too sweet: granola, oatmeal (steel cut oats), whole grain cereal, etc.	Primarily	
	Grains without gluten: amaranth, buckwheat, millet, oats, quinoa, sorghum, teff	Primarily	
	Pasta: made from black beans, buckwheat, or quinoa. Should not contain wheat (any variety), tapioca or rice flour.	Primarily	
	Rice: basmati rice (preferably brown), black rice, brown rice, red rice, wild rice. Avoid white rice.	Primarily	

Area	Foods	Eat	Note
Nuts and Seeds			
Choose unsalted or low-salt varieties that are raw or dry roasted. Store seeds in the freezer.			
	Almonds	Limited	
	Brazil nuts: nuts grown in Brazil and sold unshelled contain more selenium. Either take a selenium supplement OR eat up to 6 Brazil nuts sold shelled or 3 nuts sold unshelled each day.	Limited	
	Cashews	Limited	
	Chia seeds	Limited	
	Flaxseeds Buy whole flaxseeds and grind just before using; whole flaxseeds may pass through the digestive tract without providing benefit.	Limited	Omega-3
	Hazel nuts	Limited	
	Hemp seeds	Limited	
	Macadamia nuts	Limited	
	Pecans	Limited	
	Pistachios	Limited	
	Pumpkin seeds	Limited	
	Sesame seeds	Limited	
	Sunflower seeds	Limited	
	Walnuts	Limited	Omega-3
Snacks			
	Chocolate: dark chocolate with at least 70% cacao content. Dark chocolate has more flavonoids than milk chocolate.	Limited	
	Coconut: flakes, shredded	Primarily	
	Crackers (without gluten): oat, rice, seed crackers	Limited	

Area	Foods	Eat	Note
	Dried fruits: apricots, blueberries, cherries, cranberries (reduced sugar), currants, figs, prunes, raisins, etc.	Limited	FODMAP
	Flatbread: high fiber gluten-free flatbread	Limited	
	Goji berries	Limited	
	Tortillas made from corn, not wheat.	Limited	
Oils			
	Avocado oil	Limited	
	Coconut oil, cold pressed. Coconut oil is solid at room temperature.	Limited	
	Cocoa butter	Limited	
	Flaxseed oil Use for dressings, not cooking.	Limited	Omega-3
	Macadamia oil	Limited	
	Olive oil, extra-virgin	Limited	
	Sesame oil, roasted. Use for flavoring and dressings, not cooking.	Limited	
	Walnut oil: plain or roasted	Limited	Omega-3
Herbs and Spices			
	Herbs: dried basil, dill, oregano, parsley, rosemary, thyme, etc.	Primarily	
	Honey	Rarely	FODMAP
	Maple syrup, the real stuff, check the ingredient list.	Limited	
	Sugar	Limited	
Beverages			
	Cocoa: unsweetened raw cocoa powder. Not Dutch or alkalized cocoa.	Primarily	
	Coconut water, unsweetened	Primarily	
	Coffee	Primarily	
	Masala chai or Chai tea bags or unsweetened concentrate	Primarily	

Area	Foods	Eat	Note
	Teas: black tea, ginger, green tea, jasmine tea, oolong tea, rooibos tea, white tea; herbal teas	Primarily	
	Wine: red wine	Limited	

Convenience Foods

Area	Foods	Eat	Note
	Precooked beets, brown rice, grain mixtures (gluten free), lentils, polenta, quinoa, etc. May be refrigerated or shelf-stable; check sodium content, especially on flavored varieties.	Limited	
	Prepared vegetables or salad ingredients that are cleaned, chopped, and ready to eat or cook. Skip the croutons, cheese, and dressings made using unhealthy fats.	Primarily	
	Veggie burgers: look for burgers made from beans, soy and vegetables; check the sodium content.	Limited	

Condiments

Area	Foods	Eat	Note
	Chili sauce, hot sauce, pepper sauce, etc.	Limited	
	Juices: lemon, lime, or orange juice	Primarily	
	Ketchup, no salt variety	Limited	
	Mayonnaise	Rarely	
	Mustard	Limited	
	Salad dressing made with olive oil or other healthy fats, and not too much sodium or sweetener.	Limited	
	Salsa, enchilada sauce, taco sauce, etc.	Limited	
	Sauces in a variety of favorite tastes. Use sparingly, many sauces are high in salt or sugar, and may contain gluten.	Limited	

Area	Foods	Eat	Note
	Soy sauce or tamari. Use sparingly, even 'less-sodium' soy sauce is high in salt; most soy sauce or shoyu contains wheat but gluten-free versions are available.	Limited	
	Spreads: caponata, confit (vegetable), pesto, tapenade, etc. Check salt content.	Limited	
	Vinegars with different flavors: apple cider vinegar, balsamic vinegar, champagne vinegar, red wine vinegar, sherry vinegar, truffle vinegar, etc.	Primarily	
	Wine for cooking such as Madeira, sherry, etc. Avoid cooking wine containing added salt.	Limited	
	Worcestershire sauce is gluten free, vegetarian versions are available.	Limited	

Ingredients to Avoid

Avoid, or eat as little as possible, of foods containing ingredients shown in the list below for the reason shown in the right column. Reasons are defined in Chapter 4 and include: food additives, artificial sweeteners, grains/gluten, soy (unfermented soy), sugars (all types), and undesirable fats.

Ingredient	Reason
Acesulfame K, Ace K	Artificial Sweetener
Agave nectar	Sugars
All-purpose flour	Grains/Gluten
Aspartame	Artificial Sweetener
Autolyzed yeast	Additive
Barley	Grains/Gluten
Beet sugar	Sugars
Bread or bread crumbs	Grains/Gluten
Brown rice syrup	Sugars
Brown sugar	Sugars
Bulgur	Grains/Gluten
Cane juice	Sugars
Cane sugar	Sugars
Canola oil	Undesirable Fats
Caramel	Sugars

Ingredient	Reason
Carrageenan	Additive
Cereal extract	Grains/Gluten
Coconut sugar	Sugars
Confectioner's sugar	Sugars
Corn oil	Undesirable Fats
Corn sugar	Sugars
Corn syrup	Sugars
Cottonseed oil	Undesirable Fats
Couscous	Grains/Gluten
Cracker meal	Grains/Gluten
Date sugar	Sugars
Dextrose	Sugars
Durum wheat	Grains/Gluten
Edamame	Soy
Einkorn	Grains/Gluten
Emmer	Grains/Gluten
Enriched flour	Grains/Gluten
Farina	Grains/Gluten
Farro	Grains/Gluten
Flour	Grains/Gluten
Food starch	Grains/Gluten
Fructose	Sugars
Fruit sugar	Sugars
Fu	Grains/Gluten
Glucose	Sugars
Gluten	Grains/Gluten
Graham, graham flour	Grains/Gluten
Grape seed oil, Grapeseed oil	Undesirable Fats
High gluten flour	Grains/Gluten
High protein flour	Grains/Gluten
High-fructose corn syrup	Sugars

Ingredient	Reason
Honey	Sugars
Hydrogenated starch hydrolysates (HSH)	Artificial Sweetener
Hydrogenated oils (any type)	Undesirable Fats
Hydrolyzed vegetable protein	Soy
Isomalt	Artificial Sweetener
Kamut	Grains/Gluten
Lactitol	Artificial Sweetener
Lactose	Sugars
Levulose	Sugars
Maltitol	Artificial Sweetener
Malt syrup	Sugars
Malt	Grains/Gluten
Maltodextrin	Sugars
Maltose	Sugars
Mannitol	Artificial Sweetener
Maple sugar	Sugars
Maple syrup	Sugars
Margarine	Undesirable Fats
Matzo, matzoh, matzah, or matza	Grains/Gluten
Milk sugar	Sugars
Modified starch	Grains/Gluten
Molasses	Sugars
Mono-oleoylglycerol (MOG)	Additive
Monosodium glutamate (MSG)	Additive
Noodles	Grains/Gluten
Palm or palm kernel oil	Undesirable Fats
Partially hydrogenated oil (any)	Undesirable Fats
Pasta	Grains/Gluten
Pastry flour	Grains/Gluten
Pearled barley	Grains/Gluten
Potato starch	Sugars

Ingredient	Reason
Powdered sugar	Sugars
Rapeseed oil	Undesirable Fats
Raw sugar	Sugars
Rye	Grains/Gluten
Saccharin	Artificial Sweetener
Safflower oil	Undesirable Fats
Seitan	Grains/Gluten
Self-rising flour	Grains/Gluten
Semolina	Grains/Gluten
Shortening	Undesirable Fats
Sodium benzoate	Additive
Sodium sulfite	Additive
Sorbitol	Artificial Sweeter
Sorghum syrup	Sugars
Soy isolate	Soy
Soy protein, Soy protein isolate	Soy
Soybean oil	Undesirable Fats
Spelt	Grains/Gluten
Sprouted wheat	Grains/Gluten
Stone ground flour	Grains/Gluten
Sucanat	Sugars
Sucralose	Artificial Sweetener
Sucrose	Sugars
Sugar cane syrup	Sugars
Sunflower oil	Undesirable Fats
Tabbouleh	Grains/Gluten
Table sugar	Sugars
Tapioca starch	Sugars
Textured soy protein	Soy
Texturized vegetable protein	Soy
Tofu (unfermented)	Soy

Ingredient	Reason
Triticale	Grains/Gluten
Triticum	Grains/Gluten
Turbinado, Turbinado sugar	Sugars
Unbleached flour	Grains/Gluten
Vital gluten, vital wheat gluten	Grains/Gluten
Wheat berries	Grains/Gluten
Wheat bran	Grains/Gluten
Wheat germ, wheat germ oil	Grains/Gluten
Wheat gluten	Grains/Gluten
Wheat protein isolate	Grains/Gluten
Wheat sprouts	Grains/Gluten
Wheat starch	Grains/Gluten
White flour	Grains/Gluten
Whole wheat, whole-wheat flour	Grains/Gluten
Xylitol	Artificial Sweetener
Yeast extract	Additive

Diagnosis and Care Considerations

This appendix covers risk factors for developing lymphedema or lipedema, factors that distinguish lymphedema from lipedema, information on treatment and other health care considerations for each condition.

Risk Factors

Risk factors for lymphedema and lipedema include:

- Family history of lymphedema or lipedema, chronic swelling of the feet or legs, larger legs and hips, or abnormal fat on the upper arms (especially in women). Genetic factors for lipedema can be inherited from the father's family, even if he does not have lipedema.

- Cancer and cancer treatment, especially breast cancer (arm, breast, or truncal edema), cancers of the reproductive organs (genital, lower extremity lymphedema), head and neck cancer (head and neck lymphedema), and melanomas.

- Obesity: for adults is a BMI of 30 or more, for children and teens obesity is a BMI equal or greater than the 95th percentile norms for their age and sex. See www.cdc.gov under Healthy Weight for BMI calculators and norms.

- Liver disease including non-alcoholic fatty liver disease (NAFLD), nonalcoholic steatohepatitis (NASH), or cirrhosis of the liver. Most obese adults and many obese children have NAFLD, as do some people of normal weight.

- Diabetes or pre-diabetes (metabolic syndrome).

- High blood pressure (hypertension).

- Cardiac conditions, especially congestive heart failure (CHF).

- Chronic venous insufficiency (CVI) or varicose veins.

- Vein stripping for cardiac bypass surgery or venous ablation.

- Lymphatic system damage from injuries, burns, chronic pressure, surgery, radiation, etc.

Lipedema vs. Lymphedema

Table C-1 (page 256) and Table C-2 (page 257) highlight factors that distinguish lymphedema from lipedema.

Keep in mind that it is possible to have both lymphedema, lipedema, and obesity, see the photos in Appendix D for examples. Combinations of lipedema or lymphedema with less common adipose tissue disorders, such as Dercum's disease or multiple symmetric lipomatosis, are also possibilities.

Lymphedema Treatment

Lymphedema treatment and home care focus on slowing the progression of the condition and reducing infection risk by minimizing stagnant fluid and reducing the size of the affected area.

Complex Decongestive Therapy (CDT) for lymphedema includes:

- Skin care to maintain an effective barrier against infectious organisms.

- Lymphatic drainage by skin manipulation—Manual Lymph Drainage (MLD) or Simple Lymph Drainage (SLD)—or pump therapy (intermittent pneumatic compression).

- Compression using special bandages or garments to reduce swelling and prevent swelling from increasing.

- Exercise moves the skeletal muscles which increases the pumping action of the lymphatic system, stimulates blood circulation, and improves digestive function. Diaphragmatic breathing also stimulates the pumping action of the central lymphatic vessels.

Other Lymphedema Health Care Considerations

Lymphedema is stressful and many people with lymphedema have multiple sources of stress. Chronic stress combined with a high sugar/fat diet results in significantly more abdominal fat and increased insulin resistance than does poor diet alone [161].

People with lymphedema can become trapped in a cycle of increasing weight and isolation coupled with declining health and quality of life. Breaking this cycle may require:

- Training on healthier food choices (as outlined here).

- Practical support for buying and preparing healthier foods.

- Stress reduction and eating awareness training using techniques from mindfulness, positive psychology, cognitive-behavioral therapy, etc.

- Social support for healthy eating, increasing activity, exercise, and engagement.

The eating pattern outlined here will typically result in noticeable improvement within six weeks. Weight loss can improve existing lymphedema [162]. Risk of developing lymphedema increases with body mass and can be reduced by weight loss [163].

In addition, it may be appropriate to:

- Test for gluten sensitivity and celiac disease before reducing gluten if there are either symptoms: a history of stomach pain, gas and bloating, diarrhea, weight gain or loss, anemia or other nutrient deficiencies, bone or joint pain [164]; or risk factors: Turner syndrome, family members with celiac disease or gluten sensitivity, autoimmune thyroid disease, type 1 diabetes, or other autoimmune diseases.

- Evaluate patients with wounds or skin ulcers for nutritional deficiencies, even if they are overweight or obese, and especially after bariatric surgery, which can decrease nutrient absorption. Additional protein, vitamins C and A, and zinc may be needed to support healing [165].

- Monitor and adjust medications for other conditions—such as diabetes, hypertension, or heart failure—as needed during eating pattern changes.

Table C-1: Signs by Body Area

Area	Lymphedema	Lipedema
Head and Neck	May have swelling, rarely symmetrical	Spared initially; abnormal scalp fat with a spongy feel in Stage 4
Arms	Swelling, then fat, rarely symmetrical	Symmetrical nodular fat on triceps, biceps, forearm
Hands	Swelling, then fat	Spared initially; fat at the base of the thumb and between the knuckles in Stage 4
Breasts	Localized edema	Can be edematous if overweight
Abdomen	Swelling, fat, panniculus	Swelling, fat below umbilicus initially, later above umbilicus; panniculus if overweight
Trunk	Localized edema	Increased fat, localized edema in later stages
Genitals	May swell	Swell in later stages
Legs	Swelling, then fat, rarely symmetrical	Symmetrical fat initially; fatty extrusions especially around the knees in Stage 2 and 3
Feet and Toes	Swelling, then fat, rarely symmetrical	Spared initially (harem pants), fat in Stage 4

Table C-2: Lymphedema vs. Lipedema

Characteristic	Lymphedema	Lipedema
Fat distribution	Rarely symmetrical	Symmetrical
Fat texture	Normal	Small nodules initially, with larger nodules later
Abnormal fat locations	Feet and legs, arm, trunk	Legs (hip to ankle) and/or arms, scalp in Stage 4
Onset	Birth, puberty, or later	Puberty, by third decade
Sex predominance	Both Sexes	Mostly Female
Painful fat	No, may have pain from swelling, tight skin	Yes, touch sensitive, chronic pain
Broken blood vessels	Rare	Common, bruises easily
Pitting edema	Pitting in early stages; becomes non-pitting later	Minimal pitting
Leg swelling progression	Swelling increases from the feet up or trunk down	Stops at ankle and feet are spared initially; feet swell in Stage 4

- Tightly control glucose levels in type 2 diabetes to minimize abnormal fat accumulation, inflammation, and other effects of excess glucose and insulin.

- Address other issues that might accompany lymphedema such as insomnia, chronic pain, depression, anxiety, eating disorders, and body image concerns.

- Review medications for possible side effects that include swelling and weight gain. Analgesics and many medications of other types can contribute to swelling including drugs for diabetes, hypertension, arrhythmia, preventing blood clots and stroke (anticoagulants), cholesterol, chemotherapy, and depression.

- Use prebiotics (see "Inulin" on page 87) and probiotics to maintain healthy gut microbes during and following antibiotic treatment to reduce the risk of weight gain, diarrhea, and other antibiotic side effects [166].

Lipedema Treatment

Treatment for lipedema is essentially the same as lymphedema treatment and should start early, without waiting for visible swelling (edema) to develop. Lipedema fat can be very touch sensitive and may require very gentle treatment or treatment modifications. Pain and touch sensitivity typically decreases with compression, MLD, and careful pump treatment (intermittent pneumatic compression).

There are women with lipedema who have achieved and maintained a normal body profile and our recommendations incorporate lessons from their experiences. We have seen slow, gradual, fat loss in women with lipedema on a whole food plant based diet rich in omega-3 fats and rainbow-colored vegetables and fruits.

Other Lipedema Health Care Considerations

Women with lipedema are likely to have other health issues including:

- Thyroid abnormalities

- High blood pressure (hypertension)

- Nutritional deficiencies, especially Vitamin B12, Vitamin D and iron.

- Orthopedic issues including joint hypermobility, Ehlers-Danlos syndrome hypermobility type, flat feet, gait issues, knee problems, and arthritis.

- Psychological issues including depression or anxiety

- Fibromyalgia

- Diabetes or pre-diabetes (metabolic syndrome)

- Migraines

- Dysmenorrhea, endometriosis, polycystic ovary syndrome, ovarian cysts

- Digestive issues such as bloating, constipation, low gut motility, trouble digesting meats or fats, etc.

- Dercum's disease (adiposis dolorosa)

It may be appropriate to:

- Monitor thyroid levels and replace thyroid hormone when hypothyroidism is present to minimize weight gain.

- Minimize added estrogens from contraceptive pills or implants. IUDs with estrogen do not appear to impact lipedema.

- Avoid high dose hormone replacement therapy after the menopause. It is unclear what effect hormone replacement therapy has on lipedema fat during this phase of life.

- Avoid topical estrogens other than vaginal creams.

Appendix **D:**

Example Photos

Photo groupings:

Arms

Fig D-1: Lymphedema Stage I, right arm	Fig D-2: Lymphedema Stage I, left arm
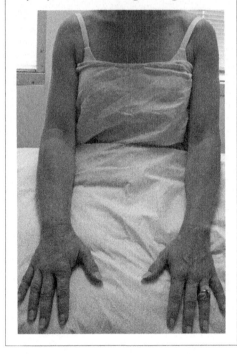	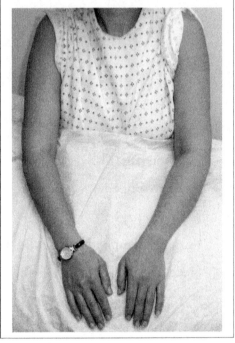

Fig D-3:
Lymphedema Stage II, right arm

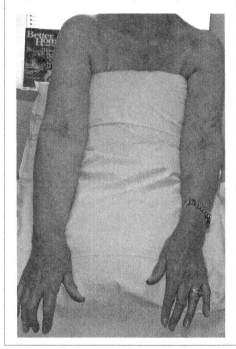

Fig D-4:
Lymphedema Stage II, right arm

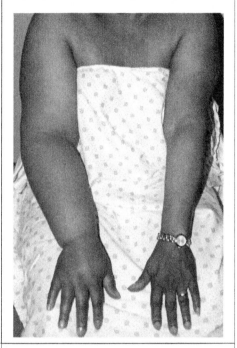

Fig D-5:
Lymphedema Stage III, right arm

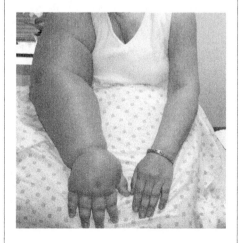

Fig D-6:
Lymphedema Stage III, right arm

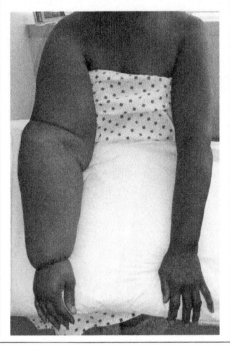

Fig D-7:
Arm Lipedema Stage 2, Type IV

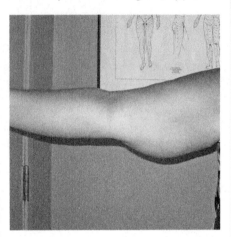

Fig D-8:
Arm Lipedema Stage 2, Type IV

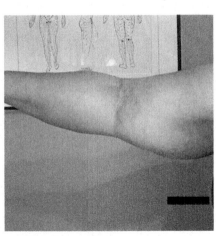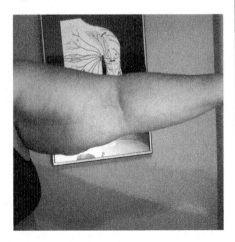

Legs

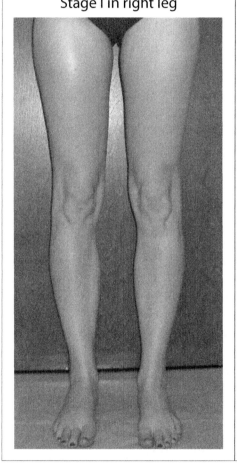

**Fig D-9:
Primary Lymphedema
Stage I in right leg**

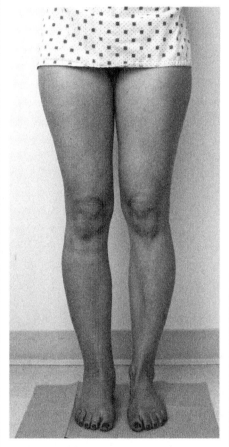

**Fig D-10:
Primary Lymphedema Stage I**

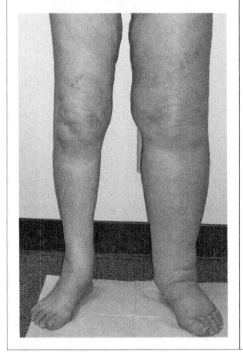

Fig D-11:
Secondary Lymphedema Stage II
in left leg

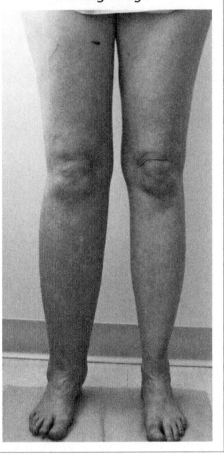

Fig D-12:
Secondary Lymphedema Stage II
in right leg

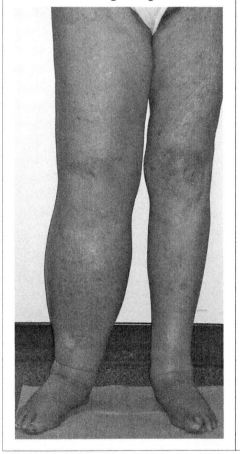

Fig D-13:
Primary Lymphedema Stage III
in right leg

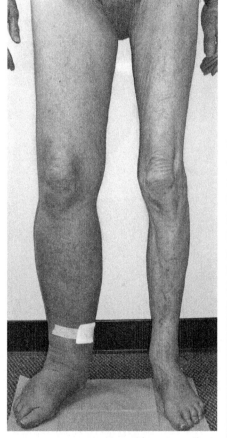

Fig D-14:
Lymphedema Stage III
in right leg

Fig D-15:
Lymphedema Stage III
in left leg

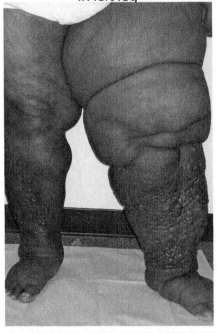

Fig D-16:
Primary Lymphedema Stage III
both legs

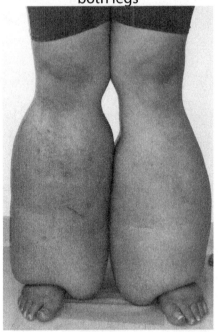

Fig D-17:
Lymphedema Stage III
both legs

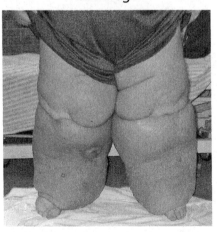

Fig D-18:
Primary Lymphedema Stage II
with abdominal panniculus

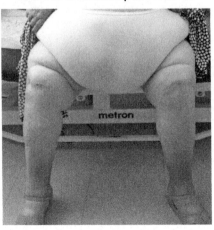

Fig D-19:
Lipedema Stage 1, Type III

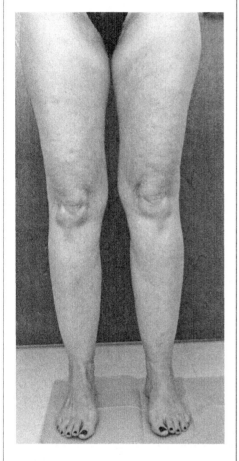

Fig D-20:
Lipedema Stage 1, Type II

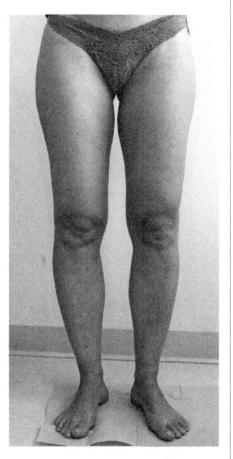

Fig D-21:
Lipedema Stage 1, Type III

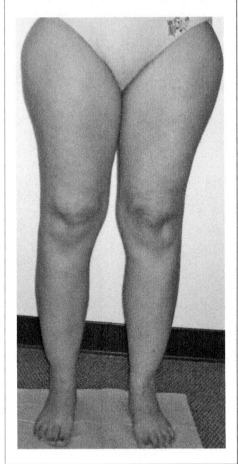

Fig D-22:
Primary Lymphedema Stage II
and Lipedema Stage 1, Type I

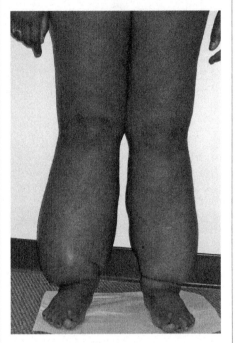

Fig D-23:
Lipedema Stage 2, Type III,
with ankle cuff

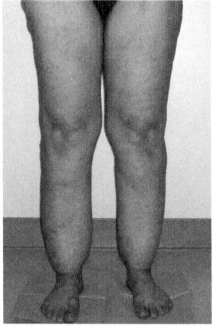

Fig D-25:
Lipedema Stage 2, Type III,
feet unaffected

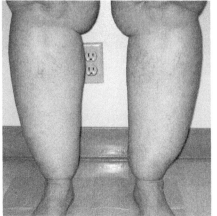

Fig D-24:
Lipedema Stage 2, Type III,
with ankle cuff

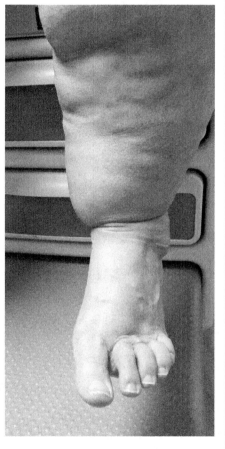

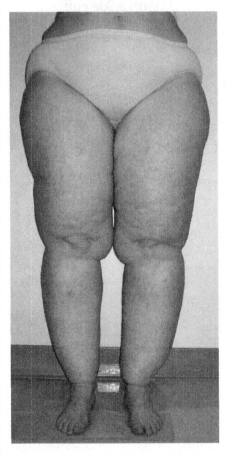

Fig D-26:
Lipedema Stage 2, Type III

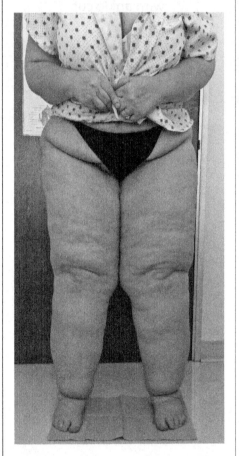

Fig D-27:
Lipedema Stage 3, Type III

Fig D-28:
Lipedema Stage 3, Type III

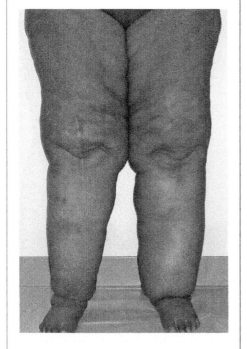

Fig D-29:
Lipedema Stage 4, Type III

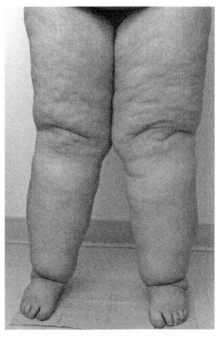

Fig D-30:
Lipedema Stage 4, Type III legs,
Type V Lipolymphedema

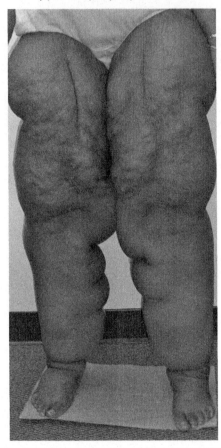

Fig D-31:
Lipedema Stage 4, Type III

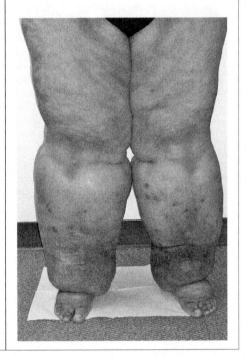

Phlebolymphedema

Fig D-32: Phlebolymphedema Stage I both legs

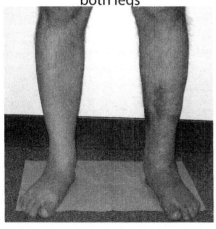

Fig D-33: Phlebolymphedema Stage II right leg, Stage I left leg

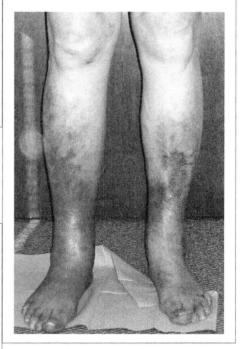

Fig D-34: Phlebolymphedema Stage II, after wound treatment

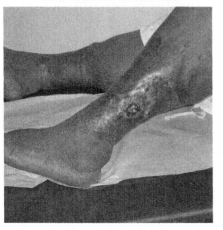

Fig D-35:
Lipedema Stage 3, Type II,
with venous disease and obesity

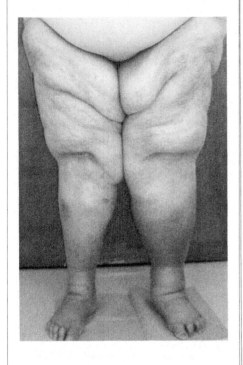

Fig D-36:
Phlebolymphedema Stage III,
before and after treatment

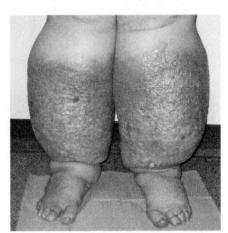

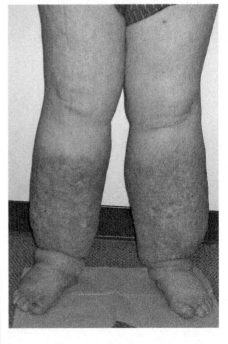

Body

Fig D-37:
Lipedema Stage 1, Type III

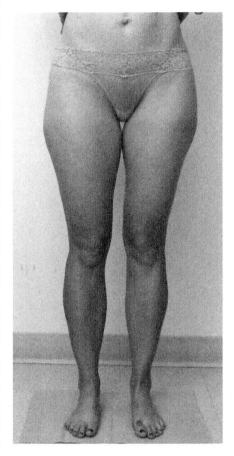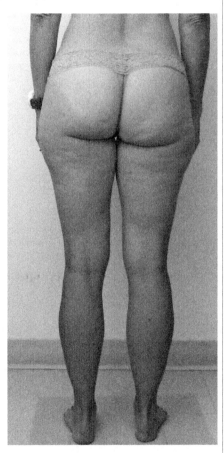

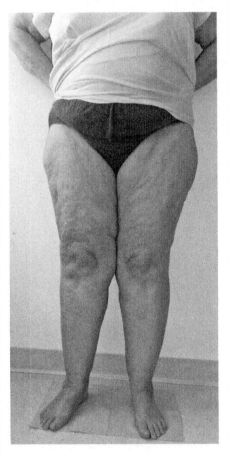

Fig D-38:
Lipedema Stage 2, Type III

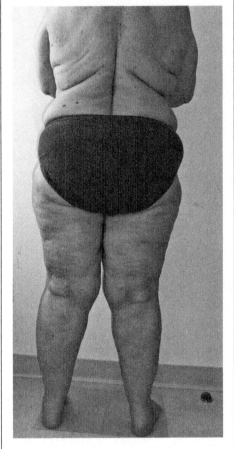

Fig D-39:
Lipedema Stage 2, Type III

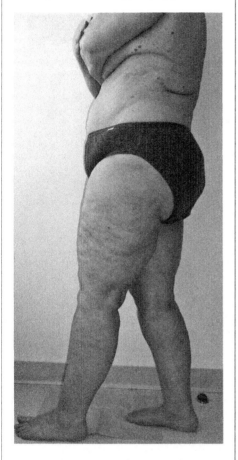

Fig D-40:
Lipedema Stage 2, Type III

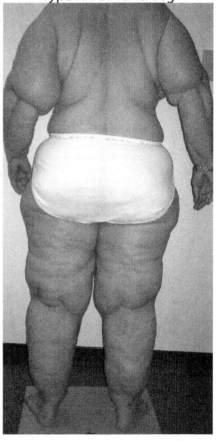

Fig D-41:
Lipedema Stage 3, Type III legs,
Type IV Arm and Leg

Fig D-42:
Lipedema Stage 3, Type IV, with obesity

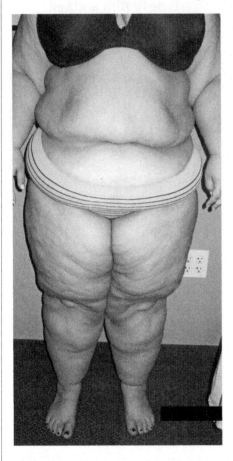 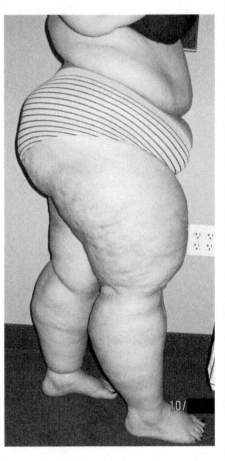

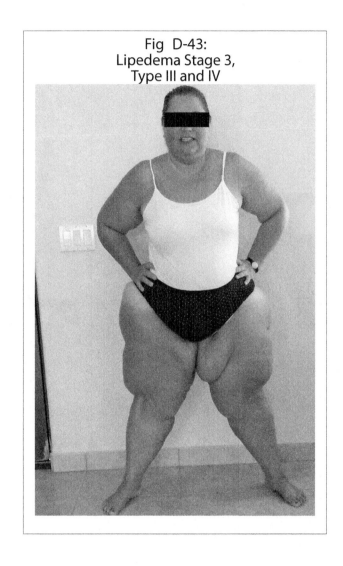

Fig D-43:
Lipedema Stage 3,
Type III and IV

Primary Lymphedema in Children

Fig D-44: Infant with Primary Lymphedema	Fig D-45: Child with Milroy Disease
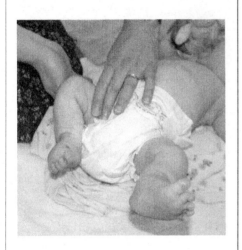	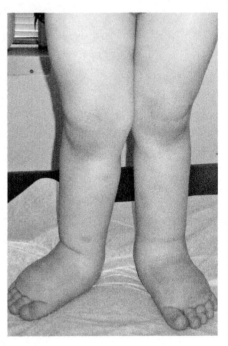

Head and Neck Lymphedema

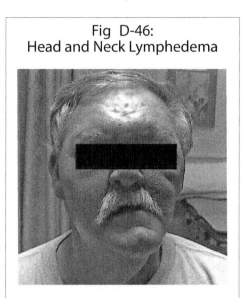

Fig D-46:
Head and Neck Lymphedema

Lymphedema and Lipedema

Books:

- **Living Well With Lymphedema** by Ann Ehrlich, Alma Vinjé-Harrewijn, PT, CLT-LANA & Elizabeth McMahon, PhD (Lymph Notes, 2005). Lymphedema patient's handbook.

- **Lymphedema Caregiver's Guide** by Mary Kathleen Kearse, PT, CLT-LANA, Elizabeth McMahon, PhD, & Ann Ehrlich (Lymph Notes, 2009). How to provide or arrange home-care.

- **Overcoming the Emotional Challenges of Lymphedema** by Elizabeth McMahon, PhD (Lymph Notes, 2005).

- **Voices of Lymphedema** edited by Ann Ehrlich & Elizabeth McMahon, PhD (Lymph Notes, 2007). Inspirational teaching stories by people with lymphedema or lipedema and therapists.

- **100 Questions & Answers About Lymphedema** by Saskia R.J. Thiadens, Paula J. Stewart, Nicole L. Stout (Jones & Bartlett Publishers, 2009).

Websites and organizations:

- American Lymphedema Framework Project www.alfp.org

- Canadian Lymphedema Framework www.canadalymph.ca

- Fat Disorders Research Society www.fatdisorders.org.

- International Lymphoedema Framework www.lympho.org

- Lymph Notes www.LymphNotes.com. Online community, resource directory, and practical information.

- Lymphatic Education & Research Network www.lymphaticnetwork.org

- National Lymphedema Network (NLN) www.lymphnet.org.

Weight and Nutrition

- Centers for Disease Control (CDC) has online BMI calculators, information on weight norms for different ages and other useful resources under Healthy Weight, see www.cdc.gov.

- USDA Supertracker has online tools for evaluating the nutritional content of foods, food and activity tracking, and much more, see www.supertracker.usda.gov.

Healthy Recipes

For meal plans, recipes, and practical tips for changing to a lower carbohydrate eating pattern see books by William Davis, MD: **Wheat Belly, Wheat Belly Cookbook,** and the **Wheat Belly 30-Minute (Or Less!) Cookbook**. Our recommended eating pattern started from the Wheat Belly list with many changes include limiting salt, soy, and animal products.

Children:

- **The Good Gut** by Justin and Erica Sonnenburg (Penguin Press, 2015). Parents and Stanford pathologists provide practical advice and recipes tested on their children.

- **Nom Nom Paleo** by Michelle Tam and Henry Fong (Andrews Mc-Meel Publishing, 2013). Wide variety of child tested recipes in a pretty book; paleo can be more meat-centric than our recommendations.

Microbiota

Follow Your Gut by Rob Knight (Simon & Schuster/TED. 2015). Concise intro to the role of microbes in health and disease. Rob Knight is a Professor of Pediatrics and Computer Science & Engineering and Director of the

Microbiome Initiative at UCSD. He is cofounder of the American Gut Project and the Earth Microbiome Project.

Missing Microbes by Martin J. Blaser, MD (Henry Holt and Co. 2015). How antibiotics and our gut microbes are affecting our health and weight.

Nutrition and Digestive Health

How Not to Die by Michael Greger, MD, and Gene Stone (Flatiron Books, 2015). Rigorous yet readable information on the scientific evidence supporting plant-based food choices and food choices to help heal or prevent chronic diseases (including diabetes, heart disease, and liver disease) that are leading causes of death.

Proteinaholic by Garth Davis, MD and Howard Jacobson(HarperOne, 2015). A weight loss surgeon dissects our obsession with animal-based protein, why meat is unnecessary and how it is detrimental to our health.

Gluten Freedom by Alessio Fasano, MD (Wiley 2014) or his **Clinical Guide to Gluten Disorders** (LWW 2013). The latest information on diagnosis and treatment for gluten sensitivity and celiac disease.

Celiac Disease by Peter Green, MD, and Rory Jones (William Morrow Paperbacks, 2010).

Fat Chance by Robert H. Lustig, MD (Plume 2013). The toxic effects of sugars and fructose on the central nervous system and metabolism explained by a pediatrician and obesity researcher from UCSF.

The Inside Tract by Gerard E. Mullin, MD (Rodale Books, 2011). Practical information on understanding and overcoming gastrointestinal conditions from an integrative medicine specialist at Johns Hopkins University.

Behavior Change

Disease-Proof by David L. Katz, MD (Plume, 2014). Katz has very good material on changing eating habits (including some we have adapted) based on his research at Yale.

The PlantPlus Diet Solution by Joan Borysenko PhD (Hay House, Inc., 2014). More good information on the process of changing eating habits.

Mindfulness and Meditation

Lovingkindness by Sharon Salzberg (Shambhala 2008).

Full Catastrophe Living by John Kabat-Zinn, PhD (Dell Publishing, 1990).

The Relaxation and Stress Reduction Workbook, 5th Ed by Martha Davis, PhD, Elizabeth Eshelman, MSW, and Matthew McKay, PhD (New Harbinger Publications, 2000).

Mindful Eating Training (www.mindfuleatingtraining.com) coaching and professional training in person, by phone or webinar; also retreats.

Eating Disorders

Overcoming Binge Eating by Christopher Fairburn, MD (Guilford Press, 1995).

Overcoming Bulimia by Randi McCabe, PhD, Traci McFarlane, PhD, and Marion Olmstead, PhD (New Harbinger Publications, 2004).

www.womenshealth.gov and www.girlshealth.gov websites provide information on eating patterns, obesity, and other health issues from the US Department of Health and Human Services.

References

1   Mauras N, et al. Estrogens and their genotoxic metabolites are increased in obese prepubertal girls. J Clin Endocrinol Metab. 2015 Apr 9:jc20151495. www.ncbi.nlm.nih.gov/pubmed/25856214

2   Anderson EL, et al. The Prevalence of Non-Alcoholic Fatty Liver Disease in Children and Adolescents: A Systematic Review and Meta-Analysis. PLoS One. 2015 Oct 29;10(10):e0140908. www.ncbi.nlm.nih.gov/pubmed/26512983

3   International Society of Lymphology. The diagnosis and treatment of peripheral lymphedema. Consensus document of the International Society of Lymphology. Lymphology 2003; 36(2): 84-91.

4   Herbst, KL. Rare Adipose disorders (RAD) masquerading as obesity. Acta Pharmalogica Sina 2012 33:155-172. www.ncbi.nlm.nih.gov/pubmed/22301856

5   MacDonald, J.M. et al "Lymphedema, Lipedema, and the Open Wound: the role of compression therapy." Surg Clin North Am. 2003 Jun:83(3):639-58. www.ncbi.nlm.nih.gov/pubmed/12822730

6   Hodson S, Eaton, S. Lipoedema management: gaps in our knowledge. Journal of Lymphoedema, 2013, Vol 8, No 1. Available from www.woundsinternational.com/media/issues/921/files/content_11243.pdf

7   Schook CC, et al. Differential diagnosis of lower extremity enlargement in pediatric patients referred with a diagnosis of lymphedema. Plast Reconstr Surg. 2011 Apr;127(4):1571-81. www.ncbi.nlm.nih.gov/pubmed/21187804

8   Herbst, KL. Rare Adipose disorders (RAD) masquerading as obesity. Acta Pharmalogica Sina 2012 33:155-172. www.ncbi.nlm.nih.gov/pubmed/22301856

9   Jones D, Min W. An overview of lymphatic vessels and their emerging role in cardiovascular disease. J Cardiovasc Dis Res 2011;2:141-52. www.ncbi.nlm.nih.gov/pubmed/22022141

10   Lee, BB et al eds. Lymphedema a concise compendium of theory and practice. Springer 2011.

11   Jones D, Min W. An overview of lymphatic vessels and their emerging role in cardiovascular disease. J Cardiovasc Dis Res 2011;2:141-52. www.ncbi.nlm.nih.gov/pubmed/22022141

12   McCray S, Parrish CR. Nutritional management of Chyle Leaks, an update. Practical Gastroenterology 2011; 35 (4): p12-32. www.practicalgastro.com/pdf/April11/McCrayArticle.pdf

13   Scallan JP, et al. Lymphatic vascular integrity is disrupted in type 2 diabetes due to impaired nitric oxide signaling. Cardiovasc Res. 2015 Jul 1;107(1):89-97. www.ncbi.nlm.nih.gov/pubmed/25852084

14   Tan B, et al. Regulatory roles for L-arginine in reducing white adipose tissue. Front Biosci (Landmark Ed). 2012 Jun 1;17:2237-46. www.ncbi.nlm.nih.gov/pubmed/22652774

15   Morris SM Jr. Arginine metabolism: boundaries of our knowledge. J Nutr. 2007 Jun;137(6 Suppl 2):1602S-1609S. www.ncbi.nlm.nih.gov/pubmed/17513435

16   Kobayashi J, et al. NO-Rich Diet for Lifestyle-Related Diseases. Nutrients. 2015 Jun 17;7(6):4911-37. www.ncbi.nlm.nih.gov/pubmed/26091235

17   Cani PD, et al. Involvement of gut microbiota in the development of low-grade inflammation and type 2 diabetes associated with obesity. Gut Microbes. 2012 Jul-Aug;3(4):279-88. Epub 2012 May 14. www.ncbi.nlm.nih.gov/pubmed/22572877

18   Musso G, et al. Obesity, diabetes, and gut microbiota: the hygiene hypothesis expanded? Diabetes Care. 2010 Oct;33(10):2277-84. www.ncbi.nlm.nih.gov/pubmed/20876708

19   Pasini E, et al. Pathogenic Gut Flora in Patients With Chronic Heart Failure. JACC Heart Fail. 2015 Dec 7. pii: S2213-1779(15)00698-8. www.ncbi.nlm.nih.gov/pubmed/26682791

20   Cordts PR, et al. Could gut-liver function derangements cause chronic venous insufficiency? Vasc Surg. 2001 Mar-Apr;35(2):107-14. www.ncbi.nlm.nih.gov/pubmed/11668378

21   Mace OJ, et al. Pharmacology and physiology of gastrointestinal enteroendocrine cells. Pharmacol Res Perspect. 2015 Aug;3(4):e00155. www.ncbi.nlm.nih.gov/pubmed/26213627

22   Veiga P, et al. Changes of the human gut microbiome induced by a fermented milk product. Sci Rep. 2014 Sep 11;4:6328. www.ncbi.nlm.nih.gov/pubmed/25209713

23   Musso G, et al. Obesity, diabetes, and gut microbiota: the hygiene hypothesis expanded? Diabetes Care. 2010 Oct;33(10):2277-84. www.ncbi.nlm.nih.gov/pubmed/20876708

24   Deopurkar R, et al. Differential effects of cream, glucose, and orange juice on inflammation, endotoxin, and the expression of Toll-like receptor-4 and suppressor of cytokine signaling-3. Diabetes Care. 2010 May;33(5):991-7. www.ncbi.nlm.nih.gov/pubmed/20067961

25   Devkota S, Chang EB. Diet-induced expansion of pathobionts in experimental colitis: implications for tailored therapies. Gut Microbes. 2013 Mar-Apr;4(2):172-4. www.ncbi.nlm.nih.gov/pubmed/23333863

26   Benoit B, et al. Pasture v. standard dairy cream in high-fat diet-fed mice: improved metabolic outcomes and stronger intestinal barrier. Br J Nutr. 2014 Aug 28;112(4):520-35. www.ncbi.nlm.nih.gov/pubmed/24932525

27   Ghanim H, et al. Orange juice neutralizes the proinflammatory effect of a high-fat, high-carbohydrate meal and prevents endotoxin increase and Toll-like receptor expression. Am J Clin Nutr. 2010 Apr;91(4):940-9. www.ncbi.nlm.nih.gov/pubmed/20200256

28   Walaszek Z, et al. Metabolism, uptake, and excretion of a D-glucaric acid salt and its potential use in cancer prevention. Cancer Detect Prev. 1997;21(2):178-90. www.ncbi.nlm.nih.gov/pubmed/9101079

29   Serena G, et al. The Role of Gluten in Celiac Disease and Type 1 Diabetes. Nutrients. 2015 Aug 26;7(9):7143-62. www.ncbi.nlm.nih.gov/pubmed/26343710

30   Catassi C, et al. Non-Celiac Gluten sensitivity: the new frontier of gluten related disorders. Nutrients. 2013 Sep 26;5(10):3839-53. www.ncbi.nlm.nih.gov/pubmed/24077239

31   El-Salhy M, et al. The relation between celiac disease, nonceliac gluten sensitivity and irritable bowel syndrome. Nutr J. 2015 Sep 7;14:92. www.ncbi.nlm.nih.gov/pubmed/26345589

32   Rashtak S, Murray JA. Celiac disease in the elderly. Gastroenterol Clin North Am. 2009 Sep;38(3):433-46. www.ncbi.nlm.nih.gov/pubmed/19699406

33   Bao F, Green PH, Bhagat G. An update on celiac disease histopathology and the road ahead. Arch Pathol Lab Med. 2012 Jul;136(7):735-45. www.ncbi.nlm.nih.gov/pubmed/22742547

34   Gravholt, C. Clinical practice in Turner syndrome. Nat Clin Pract Endocrinol Metab. 2005 Nov;1(1):41-52. www.ncbi.nlm.nih.gov/pubmed/16929365

35   Freeman, HJ and Nimmo, M. Intestinal lymphangiectasia in adults. World J Gastrointest Oncol. Feb 15, 2011; 3(2): 19–23. www.ncbi.nlm.nih.gov/pmc/articles/PMC3046182/

36   Serena G, et al. The Role of Gluten in Celiac Disease and Type 1 Diabetes. Nutrients. 2015 Aug 26;7(9):7143-62. www.ncbi.nlm.nih.gov/pubmed/26343710

37   Basaranoglu M, et al. Carbohydrate intake and nonalcoholic fatty liver disease: fructose as a weapon of mass destruction. Hepatobiliary Surg Nutr. 2015 Apr;4(2):109-16. www.ncbi.nlm.nih.gov/pubmed/26005677

38   Anderson EL, et al. The Prevalence of Non-Alcoholic Fatty Liver Disease in Children and Adolescents: A Systematic Review and Meta-Analysis. PLoS One. 2015 Oct 29;10(10):e0140908. www.ncbi.nlm.nih.gov/pubmed/26512983

39   Alexander JS, et al. Gastrointestinal lymphatics in
health and disease. Pathophysiology. 2010 Sep;17(4):315-35.
www.ncbi.nlm.nih.gov/pubmed/20022228

40   Aron-Wisnewsky J, et al. Gut microbiota and non-alcoholic fatty
liver disease: new insights. Clin Microbiol Infect. 2013 Apr;19(4):338-48.
www.ncbi.nlm.nih.gov/pubmed/23452163

41   Basaranoglu M, et al. Carbohydrate intake and nonalcoholic fatty
liver disease: fructose as a weapon of mass destruction. Hepatobiliary Surg
Nutr. 2015 Apr;4(2):109-16. www.ncbi.nlm.nih.gov/pubmed/26005677

42   Walker RW, et al. Fructose content in popular beverages made
with and without high-fructose corn syrup. Nutrition. 2014 Jul-
Aug;30(7-8):928-35. www.ncbi.nlm.nih.gov/pubmed/24985013

43   Fischer LM, et al. Dietary choline requirements of women: effects
of estrogen and genetic variation. Am J Clin Nutr. 2010 Nov;92(5):1113-9.
www.ncbi.nlm.nih.gov/pubmed/20861172

44   Green CJ, Hodson L. The influence of dietary fat on
liver fat accumulation. Nutrients. 2014 Nov 10;6(11):5018-33.
www.ncbi.nlm.nih.gov/pubmed/25389901

45   Wiig H, et al. Immune cells control skin lymphatic electrolyte
homeostasis and blood pressure. J Clin Invest. 2013 Jul 1;123(7):2803-15.
www.ncbi.nlm.nih.gov/pubmed/23722907

46   Mizuno R, et al. A High-Salt Diet Differentially Modulates
Mechanical Activity of Afferent and Efferent Collecting Lymphatics in
Murine Iliac Lymph Nodes. Lymphat Res Biol. 2015 Jun;13(2):85-92.
www.ncbi.nlm.nih.gov/pubmed/26091404

47   Bedoya SK, et al. Th17 cells in immunity and
autoimmunity. Clin Dev Immunol. 2013;2013:986789.
www.ncbi.nlm.nih.gov/pubmed/24454481

48   Lee, BB, et al eds. Lymphedema a concise compendium of theory
and practice. Springer 2011.

49   Fink AM, et al. Serum level of VEGF-D in patients
with primary lymphedema. Lymphology. 2004 Dec;37(4):185-9.
www.ncbi.nlm.nih.gov/pubmed/15693535

50   Saaristo A, et al. Insights into the molecular pathogenesis and targeted treatment of lymphedema. Ann N Y Acad Sci. 2002 Dec;979:94-110. www.ncbi.nlm.nih.gov/pubmed/12543720

51   Folkman J. Tumor angiogenesis: therapeutic implications. N Engl J Med. 1971 Nov 18; 285(21):1182-6. www.ncbi.nlm.nih.gov/pubmed/4938153

52   Campisi C, et al. Lymphedema secondary to breast cancer treatment: possibility of diagnostic and therapeutic prevention. Ann Ital Chir. 2002 Sep-Oct;73(5):493-8. www.ncbi.nlm.nih.gov/pubmed/12704989

53   Szolnoky G, et al. Lipedema is associated with increased aortic stiffness. Lymphology 45 (2012) 71-79. www.ncbi.nlm.nih.gov/pubmed/23057152

54   Jones D, Min W. An overview of lymphatic vessels and their emerging role in cardiovascular disease. J Cardiovasc Dis Res 2011;2:141-52. www.ncbi.nlm.nih.gov/pubmed/22022141

55   Galic S, et al, Adipose tissue as an endocrine organ. Mol Cell Endocrinol. 2010 Mar 25;316(2):129-39. Epub 2009 Aug 31. www.ncbi.nlm.nih.gov/pubmed/19723556

56   Jones D, Min W. An overview of lymphatic vessels and their emerging role in cardiovascular disease. J Cardiovasc Dis Res 2011;2:141-52. www.ncbi.nlm.nih.gov/pubmed/22022141

57   Carmeliet P, Jain RK. Angiogenesis in cancer and other diseases. Nature. 2000 Sep 14;407(6801):249-57. www.ncbi.nlm.nih.gov/pubmed/11001068

58   Asberg M, et al. Novel biochemical markers of psychosocial stress in women. PLoS One. 2009;4(1):e3590. Epub 2009 Jan 29. www.ncbi.nlm.nih.gov/pubmed/19177163

59   Edirisinghe I, et al. Cigarette-smoke-induced oxidative/nitrosative stress impairs VEGF- and fluid-shear-stress-mediated signaling in endothelial cells. Antioxid Redox Signal. 2010 Jun 15;12(12):1355-69. www.ncbi.nlm.nih.gov/pubmed/19929443

60   NCI. Factsheet: Angiogenesis Inhibitors. Reviewed 2011-10-07.
www.cancer.gov/cancertopics/factsheet/Therapy/angiogenesis-inhibitors

61   Boivin D, et al. Antiproliferative and antioxidant
activities of common vegetables: A comparative
study. Food Chem. 2009;112:374–80. Available from
www.chrisbeatcancer.com/wp-content/uploads/2013/01/Anti-Cancer-
Vegetables-Study.pdf

62   Li WW, et al. Tumor angiogenesis as a target for dietary
cancer prevention. J Oncol. 2012;2012:879623. Epub 2011 Sep 29.
www.ncbi.nlm.nih.gov/pubmed/21977033

63   Szel E, et al. Pathophysiological dilemmas of
lipedema. Med Hypotheses. 2014 Nov;83(5):599-606.
www.ncbi.nlm.nih.gov/pubmed/25200646

64   Suga H, et al. Adipose tissue remodeling in lipedema:
adipocyte death and concurrent regeneration. J Cutan Pathol. 2009
Dec;36(12):1293-8. www.ncbi.nlm.nih.gov/pubmed/19281484

65   Szel E, et al. Pathophysiological dilemmas of
lipedema. Med Hypotheses. 2014 Nov;83(5):599-606.
www.ncbi.nlm.nih.gov/pubmed/25200646

66   Vrtacnik P, et al. The many faces of estrogen signaling.
Biochem Med (Zagreb). 2014 Oct 15;24(3):329-42.
www.ncbi.nlm.nih.gov/pubmed/25351351

67   Szel E, et al. Pathophysiological dilemmas of
lipedema. Med Hypotheses. 2014 Nov;83(5):599-606.
www.ncbi.nlm.nih.gov/pubmed/25200646

68   Van Pelt RE, et al. Acute modulation of adipose tissue lipolysis by
intravenous estrogens. Obesity (Silver Spring). 2006 Dec;14(12):2163-72.
www.ncbi.nlm.nih.gov/pubmed/17189542

69   Tepper PG, et al. Trajectory clustering of estradiol and
follicle-stimulating hormone during the menopausal transition
among women in the Study of Women's Health across the Nation
(SWAN). J Clin Endocrinol Metab. 2012 Aug;97(8):2872-80.
www.ncbi.nlm.nih.gov/pubmed/22659249

70   Tepper PG, et al. Trajectory clustering of estradiol and follicle-stimulating hormone during the menopausal transition among women in the Study of Women's Health across the Nation (SWAN). J Clin Endocrinol Metab. 2012 Aug;97(8):2872-80. www.ncbi.nlm.nih.gov/pubmed/22659249

71   Lewis SS, et al. Select steroid hormone glucuronide metabolites can cause toll-like receptor 4 activation and enhanced pain. Brain Behav Immun. 2015 Feb;44:128-36. www.ncbi.nlm.nih.gov/pubmed/25218902

72   Braundmeier AG, et al. Individualized medicine and the microbiome in reproductive tract. Front Physiol. 2015 Apr 1;6:97. www.ncbi.nlm.nih.gov/pubmed/25883569

73   Shapira I, et al. Evolving concepts: how diet and the intestinal microbiome act as modulators of breast malignancy. ISRN Oncol. 2013 Sep 25;2013:693920. www.ncbi.nlm.nih.gov/pubmed/24187630

74   Harmon BE, et al. Oestrogen levels in serum and urine of premenopausal women eating low and high amounts of meat. Public Health Nutr. 2014 Sep;17(9):2087-93. www.ncbi.nlm.nih.gov/pubmed/24050121

75   Handa Y, et al. Estrogen concentrations in beef and human hormone-dependent cancers. Ann Oncol. 2009 Sep;20(9):1610-1. www.ncbi.nlm.nih.gov/pubmed/19628569

76   Kurzer MS. Hormonal effects of soy in premenopausal women and men. J Nutr. 2002 Mar;132(3):570S-573S. www.ncbi.nlm.nih.gov/pubmed/11880595

77   Rafii F. The role of colonic bacteria in the metabolism of the natural isoflavone daidzin to equol. Metabolites. 2015 Jan 14;5(1):56-73. www.ncbi.nlm.nih.gov/pubmed/25594250/

78   Patisaul HB, Jefferson W. The pros and cons of phytoestrogens. Front Neuroendocrinol. 2010 Oct;31(4):400-19. www.ncbi.nlm.nih.gov/pubmed/20347861/

79   Sun Q, et al. Gut microbiota metabolites of dietary lignans and risk of type 2 diabetes: a prospective investigation in two cohorts of U.S. women. Diabetes Care. 2014;37(5):1287-95. www.ncbi.nlm.nih.gov/pubmed/24550220

80   Napoli N, et al. Increased 2-hydroxylation of estrogen is associated with lower body fat and increased lean body mass in postmenopausal women. Maturitas. 2012 May;72(1):66-71. www.ncbi.nlm.nih.gov/pubmed/22385932

81   Sowers MR, et al, Selected diet and lifestyle factors are associated with estrogen metabolites in a multiracial/ethnic population of women. J Nutr. 2006 Jun;136(6):1588-95. www.ncbi.nlm.nih.gov/pubmed/16702326

82   Roy JR, et al. Estrogen-like endocrine disrupting chemicals affecting puberty in humans--a review. Med Sci Monit. 2009 Jun;15(6):RA137-45. www.ncbi.nlm.nih.gov/pubmed/19478717

83   Kurokawa S, Berry MJ. Selenium. Role of the essential metalloid in health. Met Ions Life Sci. 2013;13:499-534. www.ncbi.nlm.nih.gov/pubmed/24470102

84   Noto H, et al. Low-carbohydrate diets and all-cause mortality: a systematic review and meta-analysis of observational studies. PLoS One. 2013;8(1):e55030. www.ncbi.nlm.nih.gov/pubmed/23372809

85   Simmons AL, et al. What Are We Putting in Our Food That Is Making Us Fat? Food Additives, Contaminants, and Other Putative Contributors to Obesity. Curr Obes Rep. 2014 Jun 1;3(2):273-285. www.ncbi.nlm.nih.gov/pubmed/25045594

86   Levine JA, et al. Non-exercise activity thermogenesis: the crouching tiger hidden dragon of societal weight gain. Arterioscler Thromb Vasc Biol. 2006 Apr;26(4):729-36. www.ncbi.nlm.nih.gov/pubmed/16439708

87   de Oliveira Otto MC, et al. Dietary intake of saturated fat by food source and incident cardiovascular disease: the Multi-Ethnic Study of Atherosclerosis. Am J Clin Nutr. 2012 Aug;96(2):397-404. www.ncbi.nlm.nih.gov/pubmed/22760560

88   Boelsma E, et al. Human skin condition and its associations with nutrient concentrations in serum and diet. Am J Clin Nutr. 2003 Feb;77(2):348-55. www.ncbi.nlm.nih.gov/pubmed/12540393

89   NIH Medline Plus. Fat. Updated 2011-08-21. www.nlm.nih.gov/medlineplus/ency/article/002468.htm

90   Hayes KC, Pronczuk A. Replacing trans fat: the argument for palm oil with a cautionary note on interesterification. J Am Coll Nutr. 2010 Jun;29(3 Suppl):253S-284S. www.ncbi.nlm.nih.gov/pubmed/20823487

91   Seppanen, C.M. and A. Saari Csallany. The effect of intermittent and continuous heating of soybean oil at frying temperature on the formation of HNE and other alpha-, beta-unsaturated hydroxyaldehydes. J. Am. Oil Chem. Soc. 83 (2):121-127. http://link.springer.com/article/10.1007%2Fs11746-006-1184-0

92   Kapourchali FR, et al. The Role of Dietary Cholesterol in Lipoprotein Metabolism and Related Metabolic Abnormalities: A Mini-review. Crit Rev Food Sci Nutr. 2015 Jun 9:0. www.ncbi.nlm.nih.gov/pubmed/26055276

93   National Cancer Institute. Sources of Cholesterol among the US Population, 2005–06. Applied Research Program Web site. http://appliedresearch.cancer.gov/diet/foodsources/cholesterol/. Updated April 11, 2014. Accessed January 27, 2016.

94   Morris RC Jr et al. Relationship and interaction between sodium and potassium. J Am Coll Nutr. 2006 Jun;25(3 Suppl):262S-270S. www.ncbi.nlm.nih.gov/pubmed/16772638

95   Tappy L, Le KA. Health Effects of Fructose and Fructose-Containing Caloric Sweeteners: Where Do We Stand 10 Years After the Initial Whistle Blowings? Curr Diab Rep. 2015 Aug;15(8):627. www.ncbi.nlm.nih.gov/pubmed/26104800

96   Institute of Medicine. Dietary Reference Intakes for Energy, Carbohydrate. Fiber, Fat, Fatty Acids, Cholesterol, Protein, and Amino Acids (2002/2005). Available from www.nap.edu.

97   U.S. Department of Agriculture, Agricultural Research Service. 2014. Nutrient Intakes from Food and Beverages: Mean Amounts Consumed per Individual, by Gender and Age, What We Eat in America, NHANES 2011-2012. Available: www.ars.usda.gov/nea/bhnrc/fsrg

98   Merk & Company. The Merk Manual: Essential Fatty Acid Deficiency. June 2007. Available from www.merckmanuals.com/professional/nutritional_ disorders/undernutrition/essential_fatty_acid_deficiency.html

99 Boelsma E, et al. Human skin condition and its associations with nutrient concentrations in serum and diet. Am J Clin Nutr. 2003 Feb;77(2):348-55. www.ncbi.nlm.nih.gov/pubmed/12540393

100 Oh, Robert. "Practical Applications of Fish Oil (omega-3 fatty acids) in Primary Care." JABFP Jan-Feb 2005; V18;N1. www.ncbi.nlm.nih.gov/pubmed/15709061

101 Schwalfenbreg, Gerry. "Omega-3 fatty acids: their beneficial role in cardiovascular health." Can Fam Physician 2006;52:734-740. www.ncbi.nlm.nih.gov/pubmed/16812965

102 National Cancer Institute. Sources of Selected Fatty Acids among the US Population, 2005–06. Updated 2010-05-21. http://riskfactor.cancer.gov/diet/foodsources/fatty_acids/table2.html

103 Oh, Robert. "Practical Applications of Fish Oil (omega-3 fatty acids) in Primary Care." JABFP Jan-Feb 2005; V18;N1. www.ncbi.nlm.nih.gov/pubmed/15709061

104 Meijer K, et al. Butyrate and other short-chain fatty acids as modulators of immunity: what relevance for health? Curr Opin Clin Nutr Metab Care. 2010 Nov;13(6):715-21. www.ncbi.nlm.nih.gov/pubmed/20823773 available from www.rug.nl/research/pathology/medbiol/pdf/currentopinion_meijer2010.pdf

105 Clarke G, et al. Minireview: Gut microbiota: the neglected endocrine organ. Mol Endocrinol. 2014 Aug;28(8):1221-38. www.ncbi.nlm.nih.gov/pubmed/24892638

106 Inulin content from Moshfegh AJ, et al. Presence of inulin and oligofructose in the diets of Americans. J Nutr. 1999 Jul;129(7 Suppl):1407S-11S. www.ncbi.nlm.nih.gov/pubmed/10395608. Serving sizes from USDA National Nutrient Database http://ndb.nal.usda.gov/ndb/ accessed 2014-11-30.

107 Moshfegh AJ, et al. Presence of inulin and oligofructose in the diets of Americans. J Nutr. 1999 Jul;129(7 Suppl):1407S-11S. www.ncbi.nlm.nih.gov/pubmed/10395608

108   Per capita wheat consumption 1996, 2013 from www.ers.usda.gov/topics/crops/wheat/wheats-role-in-the-us-diet.aspx accessed 2014-12-01.

109   Falcon C M. Mapping the Genes Controlling Inulin Content in Wheat. Honors Thesis Cornell University. May 2011. Available from http://dspace.library.cornell.edu/bitstream/1813/23121/2/Falcon,%20Celeste%20-%20Research%20Honors%20Thesis.pdf

110   Suez, Jotham, et al. Artificial sweeteners induce glucose intolerance by altering the gut microbiota. Nature (2014) doi:10.1038/nature13793 www.nature.com/nature/journal/vaop/ncurrent/full/nature13793.html

111   NIH Office of Dietary Supplements. Dietary Supplement Fact Sheet: Vitamin B12 Reviewed: June 24, 2011. http://ods.od.nih.gov/factsheets/VitaminB12-HealthProfessional/

112   National Research Council. Dietary Reference Intakes for Thiamin, Riboflavin, Niacin, Vitamin B6, Folate, Vitamin B12, Pantothenic Acid, Biotin, and Choline. Washington, DC: The National Academies Press, 1998. http://books.nap.edu/catalog.php?record_id=6015

113   Kang D, et al. Vitamin B12 modulates the transcriptome of the skin microbiota in acne pathogenesis. Sci Transl Med. 2015 Jun 24;7(293):293ra103. www.ncbi.nlm.nih.gov/pubmed/26109103

114   NIH Office of Dietary Supplements. Health Professional Fact Sheets: Calcium. Available from https://ods.od.nih.gov/factsheets/Calcium-HealthProfessional/. Accessed 2016-02-18.

115   Youssef DA et al. Antimicrobial implications of vitamin D. Dermatoendocrinol. 2011 Oct;3(4):220-9. Epub 2011 Oct 1. www.ncbi.nlm.nih.gov/pubmed/22259647

116   NIH Office of Dietary Supplements. Health Professional Fact Sheets: Vitamin D. Available from https://ods.od.nih.gov/factsheets/VitaminD-HealthProfessional/ https://ods.od.nih.gov/factsheets/Calcium-HealthProfessional/. Accessed 2016-02-18.

117   NIH Office of Dietary Supplements. Health Professional Fact Sheets: Calcium. Available from https://ods.od.nih.gov/factsheets/Calcium-HealthProfessional/. Accessed 2016-02-18

118   Azoulay A, et al. Comparison of the mineral content of tap water and bottled waters. J Gen Intern Med. 2001 Mar;16(3):168-75. www.ncbi.nlm.nih.gov/pubmed/11318912

119   Rosanoff A, et al. Essential Nutrient Interactions: Does Low or Suboptimal Magnesium Status Interact with Vitamin D and/or Calcium Status? Adv Nutr. 2016 Jan 15;7(1):25-43. www.ncbi.nlm.nih.gov/pubmed/26773013

120   de Baaij JH, et al. Magnesium in man: implications for health and disease. Physiol Rev. 2015 Jan;95(1):1-46. www.ncbi.nlm.nih.gov/pubmed/25540137

121   Office of Dietary Supplements. "Dietary Supplement Fact Sheet: Magnesium." National Institutes of Health, updated 11/04/2013. Available from https://ods.od.nih.gov/factsheets/Magnesium-HealthProfessional/

122   de Baaij JH, et al. Magnesium in man: implications for health and disease. Physiol Rev. 2015 Jan;95(1):1-46. www.ncbi.nlm.nih.gov/pubmed/25540137

123   de Baaij JH, et al. Magnesium in man: implications for health and disease. Physiol Rev. 2015 Jan;95(1):1-46. www.ncbi.nlm.nih.gov/pubmed/25540137

124   Veronese N, et al. Effect of oral magnesium supplementation on physical performance in healthy elderly women involved in a weekly exercise program: a randomized controlled trial. Am J Clin Nutr. 2014 Sep;100(3):974-81. www.ncbi.nlm.nih.gov/pubmed/25008857

125   Office of Dietary Supplements. "Dietary Supplement Fact Sheet: Magnesium." National Institutes of Health, updated 11/04/2013. Available from https://ods.od.nih.gov/factsheets/Magnesium-HealthProfessional/

126   de Baaij JH, et al. Magnesium in man: implications for health and disease. Physiol Rev. 2015 Jan;95(1):1-46. www.ncbi.nlm.nih.gov/pubmed/25540137

127   Bruns F, et al. Current status of selenium and other treatments for secondary lymphedema. J Support Oncol. 2003 Jul-Aug;1(2):121-30. www.ncbi.nlm.nih.gov/pubmed/15352655

128   Office of Dietary Supplements. "Dietary Supplement Fact Sheet: Selenium." National Institutes of Health, updated: 11/12/2009. Available from http://ods.od.nih.gov/factsheets/selenium.asp.

129   Shepherd SJ, Gibson PR. Fructose malabsorption and symptoms of irritable bowel syndrome: guidelines for effective dietary management. J Am Diet Assoc. 2006 Oct;106(10):1631-9. www.ncbi.nlm.nih.gov/pubmed/17000196 available from http://sacfs.asn.au/download/SueShepherd_sarticle.pdf

130   Załęski A, et al. Butyric acid in irritable bowel syndrome. Prz Gastroenterol. 2013;8(6):350-3. www.ncbi.nlm.nih.gov/pubmed/24868283

131   Nourollahi S, et al. Bucher's Broom and Selenium Improve Lipedema: A Retrospective Case Study. Altern Integ Med 2013, 2:4.

132   Nourollahi S, et al. Bucher's Broom and Selenium Improve Lipedema: A Retrospective Case Study. Altern Integ Med 2013, 2:4.

133   Vanscheidt W, et al. Efficacy and safety of a Butcher's broom preparation (Ruscus aculeatus L. extract) compared to placebo in patients suffering from chronic venous insufficiency. Arzneimittelforschung. 2002;52(4):243-50. www.ncbi.nlm.nih.gov/pubmed/12040966

134   Sadarmin PP, Timperley J. An unusual case of Butcher's Broom precipitating diabetic ketoacidosis. J Emerg Med. 2013 Sep;45(3):e63-5. www.ncbi.nlm.nih.gov/pubmed/23849361

135   U.S. National Library of Medicine. Medline Plus: L-Arginine. www.nlm.nih.gov/medlineplus/druginfo/natural/875.html

136   Appendino G, et al. Potential role of curcumin phytosome (Meriva) in controlling the evolution of diabetic microangiopathy. A pilot study. Panminerva Med. 2011 Sep;53(3 Suppl 1):43-9. www.ncbi.nlm.nih.gov/pubmed/22108476

137   U.S. National Library of Medicine. Medline Plus: Turmeric. www.nlm.nih.gov/medlineplus/druginfo/natural/662.html

138   Badger C, et al. Benzo-pyrones for reducing and controlling lymphoedema of the limbs. Cochrane Database Syst Rev. 2004;(2):CD003140. www.ncbi.nlm.nih.gov/pubmed/15106192

139   Egert S, Rimbach G. Which sources of flavonoids: complex diets or dietary supplements? Adv Nutr. 2011 Jan;2(1):8-14. www.ncbi.nlm.nih.gov/pubmed/22211185

140   Thyagarajan-Sahu A, et al. ReishiMax, mushroom based dietary supplement, inhibits adipocyte differentiation, stimulates glucose uptake and activates AMPK. BMC Complement Altern Med. 2011 Sep 19;11:74. www.ncbi.nlm.nih.gov/pubmed/21929808

141   Calcium-D-glucarate. Altern Med Rev. 2002 Aug;7(4):336-9. www.ncbi.nlm.nih.gov/pubmed/12197785

142   Duskova M, Wald M. Orally administered proteases in aesthetic surgery. Aesthetic Plast Surg. 1999 Jan-Feb;23(1):41-4. www.ncbi.nlm.nih.gov/pubmed/10022937

143   Medline Plus. Bromelain. www.nlm.nih.gov/medlineplus/druginfo/natural/895.html

144   Maninger N, et al. Neurobiological and neuropsychiatric effects of dehydroepiandrosterone (DHEA) and DHEA sulfate (DHEAS). Front Neuroendocrinol. 2009 Jan;30(1):65-91 www.ncbi.nlm.nih.gov/pubmed/19063914

145   Adapted from Katz, David. Disease Proof. Hudson Street Press, 2013. P26.

146   Adapted from Katz, David. Disease Proof. Hudson Street Press, 2013. P29.

147   Adapted from Katz, David. Disease Proof. Hudson Street Press, 2013. P220.

148   Parts from Katz, David. Disease Proof. Hudson Street Press, 2013. P224.

149   Epictetus, Trans. Nicholas White. Handbook of Epictetus. Hackett 1983. Per http://en.wikipedia.org/wiki/Serenity_Prayer

150   Steinhausen HC. Outcome of eating disorders.
Child Adolesc Psychiatr Clin N Am. 2009 Jan;18(1):225-42.
www.ncbi.nlm.nih.gov/pubmed/19014869

151   Katz, David. Disease Proof. Hudson Street Press, 2013. P82.

152   Borysenko, Joan. The Plant Plus Diet Solution. Hay House 2014.
P184.

153   Adapted from Katz, David. Disease Proof. Hudson Street Press,
2013. P167.

154   Jaremka LM, et al. Interpersonal stressors predict ghrelin and
leptin levels in women. Psychoneuroendocrinology. 2014 Oct;48:178-88.
www.ncbi.nlm.nih.gov/pubmed/25032903

155   Katz, David. Disease Proof. Hudson Street Press, 2013. P240.

156   Adapted from Katz, David. Disease Proof. Hudson Street Press,
2013. P36.

157   Marinac CR, et al. Prolonged Nightly Fasting and
Breast Cancer Risk: Findings from NHANES (2009-2010).
Cancer Epidemiol Biomarkers Prev. 2015 May;24(5):783-9.
www.ncbi.nlm.nih.gov/pubmed/25896523

158   Marinac CR, et al. Frequency and Circadian Timing of
Eating May Influence Biomarkers of Inflammation and Insulin
Resistance Associated with Breast Cancer Risk. PLoS One. 2015 Aug
25;10(8):e0136240. www.ncbi.nlm.nih.gov/pubmed/26305095

159   Jakubowicz D, et al. Fasting Until Noon Triggers Increased
Postprandial Hyperglycemia and Impaired Insulin Response
After Lunch and Dinner in Individuals With Type 2 Diabetes: A
Randomized Clinical Trial. Diabetes Care. 2015 Oct;38(10):1820-6.
www.ncbi.nlm.nih.gov/pubmed/26220945

160   Ginsberg GL, Toal BF. "Quantitative approach for
incorporating methylmercury risks and omega-3 fatty acid benefits
in developing species-specific fish consumption advice." Environ
Health Perspect. 2009 Feb;117(2):267-75. Epub 2008 Sep 3.
www.ncbi.nlm.nih.gov/pubmed/19270798

161   Anderson EL, et al. The Prevalence of Non-Alcoholic Fatty Liver Disease in Children and Adolescents: A Systematic Review and Meta-Analysis. PLoS One. 2015 Oct 29;10(10):e0140908. www.ncbi.nlm.nih.gov/pubmed/26512983

162   Shaw C, et al. "A randomized controlled trial of weight reduction as a treatment for breast cancer-related lymphedema." Cancer 2007 Oct 15;110(8):1868-74. http://onlinelibrary.wiley.com/doi/10.1002/cncr.22994/pdf

163   Ridner SH, et al. Body mass index and breast cancer treatment-related lymphedema. Support Care Cancer. 2011 Jun;19(6):853-7. Epub 2011 Jan 16. www.ncbi.nlm.nih.gov/pubmed/21240649

164   Holtmeier W, Caspary WF. Celiac disease. Orphanet J Rare Dis. 2006 Mar 1;1:3. www.ncbi.nlm.nih.gov/pubmed/16722573

165   White-Chu EF, Conner-Kerr TA. Overview of guidelines for the prevention and treatment of venous leg ulcers: a US perspective. J Multidiscip Healthc. 2014 Feb 11;7:111-7. www.ncbi.nlm.nih.gov/pubmed/24596466

166   Hernandez E, et al. Functional consequences of microbial shifts in the human gastrointestinal tract linked to antibiotic treatment and obesity. Gut Microbes. 2013 Jul-Aug;4(4):306-15. www.ncbi.nlm.nih.gov/pubmed/23782552

Index

N

Acknowledgements

The authors would like to thank everyone involved in discussing our nutrition papers over the years.

Special thank you to:

- Linda Boyle, PT, CLT-LANA
- Laura Ehrlich, BSN, RN
- Wade Farrow, MD
- Mary Kathleen Kearse, PT, CLT-LANA
- Leslyn Keith, MS, OTR/L, CLT-LANA
- Adie MacKenzie, LMT, CLT-LANA
- Ann Myers, MD
- Sheila Ridner, PhD, RN
- Stanley Rockson, MD
- Carol Schroeder
- Katrina Schroeder, RD
- Paula Stewart, MD
- Kathryn McKillip Thrift, BS, CLT-LANA
- Joe Zuther

About the Authors

Chuck Ehrlich, MS, MBA

Chuck Ehrlich is the organizer of the lipedema study group and a medical writer for Lymph Notes. He has been studying nutrition and lymphedema since 2005. His background includes explaining many complex topics, teaching, and consulting. He received his MS from Case Western Reserve University and his MBA from University of San Francisco.

Emily Iker, MD

Emily Iker understands lymphedema on a personal level as a cancer survivor, lymphedema patient, and medical specialist. She received her MD from St. Georgia's University and advanced training in physical medicine, rehabilitation and holistic medicine. She specializes in diagnosis, management and treatment of lymphatic disorders at the Lymphedema Center in Santa Monica (www.lymphedemacenter.com).

Karen Louise Herbst, PhD, MD

Karen Herbst is an Associate Professor at University of Arizona and leader of the Treatment, Research and Education of Adipose Tissue (TREAT) Program working to better understand, diagnose, and treat adipose tissue disorders. Her research and clinical practice focus on lymphatic issues, lipedema, and other adipose tissue disorders. She is also an active fat and lymphatic disease advocate, see her blog: www.lipomadoc.org.

Linda-Anne Kahn. CMT, NCTMB, CLT-LANA, CCN

Linda-Anne Kahn is a nationally certified massage therapist and lymphedema therapist with over 30 years of experience. She has certifications as a Manual Lymph Drainage Therapist and Lymphedema Specialist from the Dr. Vodder School in Austria, the Foeldi Clinic in Germany, Drs Judith and John Casley-Smith in Australia, and the Lymphology Association of North America (LANA). She is also a certified Aromatherapist, CIDES-CO Beauty Therapist, nutritional consultant, and integrative health coach. She practices at Beauty Kliniek Day Spa and Wellness Center in San Diego (www.pamperyou.com).

Dorothy D. Sears, PhD

Dorothy Sears is an Associate Professor at University of California San Diego with a dual appointment in medicine (endocrinology and metabolism) and public health (preventive medicine). Her research specialties include obesity, diabetes, obesity-related conditions, and dietary and behavior interventions for reducing chronic disease risk. She received her PhD from Johns Hopkins University.

Mandy Kenyon, MS, RD, CSSD

Mandy Kenyon is consulting dietitian and research coordinator for the Salk Institute, Pathway Genomics, Veteran's Medical Research Foundation, and the Los Angeles County Fire Department. In addition to providing nutrition and fitness counselling, she supports several health-related research programs. She received her MS in food science and nutrition from Colorado State University.

Elizabeth McMahon, PhD

Elizabeth McMahon is a clinical psychologist in private practice and frequent speaker to patient and professional groups. Her other books include **Overcoming the Emotional Challenges of Lymphedema** and **Voices of Lymphedema**. She received her PhD from Case Western Reserve University. See www.elizabeth-mcmahon.com.

CPSIA information can be obtained
at www.ICGtesting.com
Printed in the USA
LVOW04s0749100916

504045LV00008B/401/P

9 780976 480686